ADVANCED PRAISE FOR
A LIFE UNBURDENED

Richard's book will be an inspirational guide to everyone who wants to take the lifelong journey towards health. Most especially it will be helpful for those struggling with their weight; but for everyone Richard's story will serve as a helpful guide to improving their personal health and the health of the world in which we live.

Thomas S. Cowan, M.D.
Author of *The Fourfold Path To Healing*

Richard Morris' story compels through its simplicity. In the midst of a fad-oriented society, this book illustrates how a relationship between farmer and patron can heal more successfully than all the techno-glitzy and packaged solutions society offers.

Joel Salatin, Farmer
Author of *Everything I Want To Do Is Illegal*

Morris has succeeded superbly. *A Life Unburdened* is two books in one: a deeply moving story of his battle against seemingly insurmountable odds and a treasure trove of helpful, practical hints on overcoming the physical and psychological traps that ensnare so many weight-loss hopefuls.

Anthony Colpo, Researcher
Author of *The Great Cholesterol Con*

D1358038

i

ᴀLife
Unburdened

Getting Over Weight and Getting on with My Life

Richard Morris

C O P Y R I G H T

Published by NewTrends Publishing
Washington, DC
(877) 707-1776
www.newtrendspublishing.com

First Printing, November 2005: 3,200
Second Printing, October 2007: 5,000

Printed in the United States of America

Library of Congress Control Number: 2005933912

ISBN 0-9792095-1-x
978-0-9792095-1-2

Publisher's Note: This book is not intended as a substitute for medical advice. The contents are provided with the aim of sharing the personal experiences and opinions of the author for informational purposes only. Neither the publisher nor the author shall be held liable for any consequences resulting or allegedly resulting from any action undertaken by any person reading, or following the information in this book. Consequently, neither the publisher nor the author is responsible for any condition you have, or may have in the future, that may require medical supervision. Additionally, you are advised and encouraged to confer with your health care provider regarding the undertaking of any actions or the existence of any medical conditions that affect your health.

Internet addresses, book titles, and author information were accurate up to the date of publication. Neither the publisher nor the author shall be held liable for any errors or changes that occur after the date of publication.

DEDICATION

To my wife Mary
and my daughters Stephanie and Raven

ACKNOWLEDGMENTS

In his motivational book, *Think And Grow Rich*, Napoleon Hill introduces readers to the Master Mind Principle, which states that when two or more people come together to apply their intellects toward a common goal, great things can happen. This book is a testament to the power of the Master Mind and to the enduring faith of like-minded friends, family and associates. You can never say thank you enough to the people who help you reach your goals, but you should always try.

I would like to acknowledge the nucleus of my Master Mind by saying thank you to my wife Mary and to my daughters Stephanie and Raven. Several key people provided their professional expertise and personal time to this project and made it better. They are Carol Morris, Teri Miller, Alana Sugar, CN, Sharon Wong, Katherine Czapp, Kirk Kramer and Sally Fallon.

I must also accord special recognition to the Weston A. Price Foundation and its enthusiastic members, who have dedicated themselves to providing the public with accurate information about nutrition, and to all the dedicated farmers and independent producers who work hard every day to provide families like mine with real food.

Thank you all for your assistance, your energy, and your encouragement. Finally, to Cora Morris, as always, you were right. Thank you.

Contents

Foreword

What happens when a fat man who should have been a stand-up comic loses over one hundred fifty pounds and then writes about it? You get a book that is funny, poignant, insightful, interesting, readable and inspirational.

What happens when a fat man who's failed at all the diets stops blaming his lack of willpower and figures out that all the expert advice on dieting is wrong? You get a truly practical road map to successful weight loss.

What happens when a fat man wakes up to the fact that the only way to achieve real health is to eat real food? You get stunning, inspiring life-style transformation.

A Life Unburdened is a myth-breaker. Richard Morris demolishes them one after another: the myth that eating fat makes you fat, the myth that no food is better than any other food, the myth that junk food in moderation won't hurt you, the myth that all calories are the same, the myth that no one has time to cook, the myth that losing weight will automatically make you healthy, the myth that exercise will cure disease. Morris sheds myths the way he has shed pounds, emerging as a new man from the fog of misinformation.

His program is simple. . . and absolutely radical: don't eat processed food. Ever. Eat only real food and only when you have prepared it yourself.

And what is real food? All the foods the experts have told us not to eat: butter, lard, beef, whole raw milk, eggs, liver, coconut, cream.

His message is absolutely liberating: the only way to lose weight and be healthy is to eat foods that are satisfying. Satisfying foods are foods that contain the F word—fats, old-fashioned fats, the fats our ancestors ate. Satisfying foods are foods prepared the way your grandmother made them, with soup bones and love. Satisfying foods are foods that give your body what it needs, so you're not hungry an hour later. Satisfying foods grow in gardens nearby, not monocropped furrows in far-off places. Satisfying foods come from animals that live outdoors, not in factories. Satisfying foods have not been adulterated, embalmed, emulsified, sterilized, pasteurized, irradiated, manipulated or standardized.

Morris arrives at his breathtaking epiphany by asking the right questions. Why were the members of his family getting fatter, and fatter sooner, in each generation? Why were they dying so young? Why did he keep hearing that food should be convenient? Why did dieting make him depressed and lethargic? Why did the "experts," the MDs, PhDs and RDs, keep promoting the same dietary advice when it obviously was not working?

Morris does not have a bunch of letters after his name but he has a different kind of credential—he's been there, been in the trenches. He has lived the physical and emotional agony of being fat. He has lost weight on all the diets—before gaining it all back and more. And he has achieved the supreme accomplishment of transforming himself from an obese to a normal man by making one revolutionary change: real food instead of processed food. Everything else followed from there—slow and steady weight loss, a rebirth of optimism, the end of cravings, resolution of health problems, enthusiasm for exercise, new goals, improved family life, hope for the future.

A Life Unburdened is more than just a diet book, it is a saga, and more than a saga of one man only, but of a couple and a family, a saga in which the discerning and supportive role of Richard's wife Mary emerges as an example of quiet heroism. It is a modern epic of self-transformation, one that unfolds with suspense and drama, as one suburban family replaces commercialism with wise principles. It begins in despair and ends in triumph.

Read, learn and enjoy!

Sally Fallon, President
The Weston A. Price Foundation
October, 2005

Part One
A Personal Journey

Introduction
Is today the day I die?

Is today the day I die?

This is the wrong question for a forty-three-year-old man to ask himself, but there it was again, the question that had become as much a part of my life as the squadron of pain that greeted me every morning. The persistent nightmares of drowning that left me breathless in the dark hours and the mad drumming of my heart at the slightest exertion during the day kept the specter of death with me constantly.

The source of my despair was my declining health. My life was a pond into which obesity and poor health had come crashing like a stone. The resulting ripple affected everything: my career, my family and my own self-image. I feared I would not live long enough to see my children reach adulthood.

In the Gospel of John, chapters 11 and 12, we read of Lazarus, brother of Mary and Martha. Lazarus was well-acquainted with death, having spent four days in the tomb until he miraculously rose from the grave at the spoken word of Jesus. Weighing in at over 400 pounds on my six-foot frame, I felt as though I were already dead, a walking sarcophagus, my life entombed in my own body. Who would rescue me? Who would raise me from the dead?

I was not alone. According to the Centers for Disease Control, up to two-thirds of Americans are either overweight or obese and carry an

1

increased risk of weight-related illness.

The clinical definitions of overweight and obesity are different, based on the "body mass index" or BMI. BMI is a height-weight standard sanctioned by the government. Overweight is defined as having a BMI greater than twenty-five, while a BMI greater than thirty is defined as obese. Anything above forty is considered morbidly obese. There is some disagreement among experts regarding where the threshold for these weight categories should fall. For the sake of simplicity, I shall generally use the terms overweight and obese interchangeably to refer to a person's physical state in which his weight is above a healthy level.

These days it's easy to find plenty of alarming news about America's expanding waistline and the associated health problems that come with it. Newspapers, television and the Internet are full of sobering stories about obesity-related diseases, miracle diet drugs and a never-ending stream of "fast" and "easy" weight-loss solutions. For years diet experts have been telling us how to lose weight, but somehow their advice just doesn't seem to work for most of us. Even when we do manage to lose some weight, even after all the dieting, deprivation and depression, we gain it all back. We soak up the message that our failure is proof of personal weakness and evidence of a masochistic desire to be fat. Many of us have acknowledged this explanation, even though deep down we know it isn't true.

The health problems that become part of your life when you become grossly overweight are too numerous to go into here, but I must mention one problem right off the bat, so that you can understand how my wife and I eventually found success. The problem I speak of is the rift between the tidy conclusions of weight-loss science as understood by many professionals and the messy truth of weight-gain reality, which fat people face every day.

Over the last fifteen years, as I ballooned from overweight to obese to morbidly obese, I had the sense that no one really understood what I was going through. This was especially true of the medical professionals, whose advice to "push away from the table," "eat in moderation" and "get plenty of exercise," had absolutely no connection with the real world I lived in. I couldn't push away from the table because I didn't know when I'd had enough. Eating in moderation sounded like a fine idea, but no one could explain to me how to do it without going on a binge later. And how could I get plenty of exercise when standing for more than five minutes was exhausting? Even today, despite the unprecedented attention given to the matter of obesity, the disconnect persists between what the professionals believe and what overweight people experience every day.

Many of the professionals who treat patients with weight-related illness have little first-hand knowledge of the challenges these people face. The problem is compounded when obesity is seen not as a health problem but as a moral failing. Even the concept of overeating, when generically applied to anyone who is overweight, can contribute to this disconnect, because sometimes what appears to be a problem of overeating is really a problem of undernourishment. One of the quirks of human behavior is our natural inclination to assume others see and experience life as we do. The oft-repeated phrase, "If I can do it, you can too," directed at an overweight person who clearly can't "do it," at least not in the way the speaker is suggesting, is evidence of this flaw in human behavior. There is, of course, some truth in the basic premise that people can modify their behavior and change their life. That is what this book is about, after all, but unless a health professional has walked in the shoes of his clients, is exceptionally empathetic or is highly skilled in nutrition and the behavioral sciences, he may never really be able to reach those people in a meaningful manner.

Some things are so personal and so painful that someone suffering from obesity may not even be able to tell them to his doctor. Likewise, some beliefs about nutrition and health are so deeply embedded in our behavior that we may not know ourselves why we eat and behave the way we do. How can doctors, many of whom lack sufficient training in nutrition, be of any use beyond writing prescriptions for the treatment of the disorders associated with excess weight? This becomes the usual scenario when, despite their best efforts, doctors become misers with their time in order to serve a growing number of patients. Byzantine insurance plans, the influence of the pharmaceutical industry, increased patient costs and declining levels of service have steadily chipped away at the doctor-patient relationship until doctors rarely even speak to their patients anymore.

I do not mean to imply that the medical community is of no help to overweight people. On the contrary, much of the useful advice about nutrition, weight loss and health available today comes from some able physicians, scientists and researchers, past and present. But another element, another voice is conspicuously absent from the national dialog that shapes policy on obesity and lifestyle recommendations. This voice cannot be found in the lofty towers of scientific conformity, nor between the covers of weight-loss books written by experts with "years of clinical experience dealing with overweight patients." To hear this voice, you must listen to someone who's been there, in the trenches and minefields, and in the kitchens and convenience stores, of Main Street, America, where the real battle for personal health is fought.

This book, then, is not an account of a carefully controlled double-blind placebo study conducted with overweight, nonsmoking, left handed men with a median age of thirty-five. Nor does it present theory and conjecture based on a meta-analysis of raw data extrapolated from long- term studies involving obese laboratory rats. The subject of this book is a real American family, faced with the real challenge of what to do about their declining health. It is about how we overcame obesity, clinical depression and a host of other illnesses by applying a ten-step plan. And it's about how we closed the gap between theoretical nutrition science and the everyday reality of two-for-one hamburgers . . . and how you can do the same.

THE LAZARUS PROJECT

"I want my life back." Those were the words, spoken to my wife Mary. In those words, I expressed the deepest sorrow for a life once flush with the bloom of human potential.

In June of 2003, Mary and I decided it was time to take responsibility for our health. We vowed to learn everything we could about nutrition and health and apply it to our lives. At the time, we felt like the walking dead and longed for the day we could live again. We weren't just doing this for ourselves, either. The health of our two daughters was at stake as well. It seemed fitting to call our experiment the Lazarus Project. Eighteen months later, we found ourselves, like Lazarus, risen from the metaphorical grave of a life weighted down with obesity and disease. We found that as our physical problems diminished, we grew younger in both mind and body. In no time, we found that we had more energy than we could handle. Suddenly our world seemed full of promise, and we began to realize that it really was possible to create happiness in our lives. Whether that happiness comes in the form of an improved relationship with someone you love, a better career or the courage to pursue your dreams, it can all be yours. What was at the center of this wonderful and dramatic change? Food!

Some health professionals tell us that it doesn't matter what we eat so long as we watch the calories. They tell us that all food is the same and that it is quantity, not quality, that counts in managing our weight and our health. We have discovered that this premise is simply not true. It is a lie that has condemned several members of our own family and countless others to a life of illness and an early grave. We discovered that food really does matter, more than we imagined. This simple "secret" is the foundation upon which we designed our own resurrection from illness and our escape from a life of despair.

The first section of this book, "A Personal Journey," looks back at where we were, beginning with a painfully detailed journal of what it was like for my wife and me to deal with obesity and its associated health problems on a daily basis. Later, in the chapter "Dieting in the Dark," we revisit some of the diets we've tried over the years in a stroll down diet memory lane.

The second section, "Losing Our Way," talks about the evolution of the food industry, the transition from home-cooked meals to processed convenience foods, and takes a behind-the-scenes look at how the industry influences what we eat and ultimately how healthy we are. The third section, "The Road Home," details what we learned and what we did to get over weight and get on with our lives. In the fourth section, "It's All About the Food," you'll get an insider's view of what's in my pantry and learn how to use the Total Food Index, a powerful tool to help you make better decisions about what you eat. Finally, the last section, "Rebirth," shares the story of a difficult challenge we faced that tested both our bodies and our spirits. Also in this section, we reveal the ten-step methodology we applied to change our lives forever.

Like Lazarus, we discovered that after death comes life. We want to share some of what we've learned and start you on your own journey toward getting over weight, getting on with a new life of better health and discovering your own greater potential.

Chapter One

A Day in the Life
of a Fat Man

Twenty-four hours, four hundred pounds and one Big Apple

I've read that people who lose a leg or an arm can sometimes feel a phantom pain in the missing limb. I had all of my parts thankfully, but there it was again, the faint memory of a crippling leg cramp from almost two decades ago. I remembered the pain, the extreme fatigue and, worst of all, the memory loss. . . a nearly complete blackout.

Standing on the south rim of the Grand Canyon with my wife, Mary, the memories came back, even as I took in the wonder of the canyon. Beneath the gathering clouds of an approaching storm, a sea of fantastic rock formations in brilliant hues of amber and crimson rolled to the distant horizon like an ocean of petrified waves. My eyes followed a mule train as it wound its way up the steep and twisting trail from the depths of the abyss. The trail plunged more than three thousand feet to the edge of a plateau that lay in the hazy distance a little more than six miles off. Six miles, a short distance relatively speaking, but six miles down and six miles back, into and out of the canyon, represented a level of difficulty that was an order of magnitude greater than the pleasant strolls we enjoyed back home, among the paved and gently rolling hills of suburban Virginia.

The last time we made this trip was 1986, eighteen years earlier. I was three years out of college and just twenty-six years old at the time. Newly married, I was ready to take on the world. Although I had already started to put on weight, I still had the physique of one accustomed to strenuous exercise. In those days, I could run for miles, cared little about what I ate and felt as though I would live forever. I had no idea what a tragic turn my health would take in the coming decades.

By May of 2003, I was a dead man walking. At more than four hundred pounds, I suffered from a toxic mix of obesity-related ills that included shortness of breath, sleep apnea, hypertension, aches and pains in my joints, depression, a frail immune system, asthma and other ailments too numerous to list here. Simply standing was painful, and walking more than a short distance, even on flat turf, was exhausting. Every part of my body complained of one ache or another. Bloated and ill, I had become an old man long before my time, and was haunted daily by the specter of an untimely death. I had long since mothballed dreams of hiking the canyon again.

And yet here I stood in February 2005, less than two years later, completely reborn and ready to take on one of the most challenging day hikes found anywhere in the lower forty-eight states. At two hundred fifty pounds, I was still a big man by most estimates, but the body that once carried over one hundred sixty pounds of excess fat now sported hardened muscle and an astonishingly slimmer physique. This transformation left me with the belief that given the right motivation, I really could move mountains. My new life owed much to a year's worth of newly acquired knowledge about nutrition. During the period of weight loss—all one hundred sixty pounds of it—I enjoyed some of the most delicious meals of my life. I also discovered that regular exercise isn't supposed to hurt and that the post-workout pain I suffered in college was really an early indication of a poor diet and my declining health.

Mary experienced a similar transformation, shedding fifty pounds while regaining her youthful figure and zest for life. Tomorrow we would be heading down the south rim's Bright Angel Trail for the first time in eighteen years. We had been preparing for this challenge for well over a year, but were we ready? Would we make it? Winter in the canyon is no joke, and snow was in the forecast for tomorrow. The question, "Would we make it?" kept repeating itself in my mind. As I stood there and looked out over the unforgiving landscape, I felt like an explorer about to embark on a journey into a harsh and uncompromising world. I had been to such a place before, trapped in my old life as a fat man. For those who have never been there, let me give you some idea of what it was like.

What does it feel like to be really fat? If you've never been there, it may be difficult to comprehend. A complex series of factors, both physical and emotional, combine to create an experience quite unlike anything else. You might say that the reality of being fat is so unlike anything else that fat people live in an entirely different world.

Theirs is a world where the pull of gravity exerts a greater-than-normal toll on the body. The sun is hotter, even in winter, and the air is always thinner. In a twist of bitter irony, everything is smaller in this world: cars, bathrooms, restaurant booths, even clothing seem designed to create the maximum amount of discomfort.

The chief preoccupation for the inhabitants of this world is the never-ending search for contentment. It is a search forever thwarted by an unfulfilled hunger and an unquenchable thirst. Self-control is non-existent in this part of the galaxy.

This world is littered with the corpses of failed dreams and missed opportunities. Humor comes at the price of personal dignity. Self-doubt and insecurity are constant companions, as are pain, illness and the ever-present shadow of premature death. Only the stout of heart can survive here, but no one really survives for very long. When death comes, for many it comes not a moment too soon.

6 A.M.

The buzzing in my head is the perfect accompaniment to the dull pain that throbs just behind my temples. The two sensations fuse to create an image of a large mechanical insect with a long, syringe-like stinger, drilling deep into my skull. The buzzing comes from my tormentor, a small alarm clock perched on the bedside table just beyond my reach. Like a lot of things recently, it is a new and unwelcome addition to my life. The pain in my head is quite a different matter. For the past month or so, it has visited me nearly every morning. I can't say whether it's the stress in my life or the high blood pressure that is causing the headaches, but I've grown quite accustomed to them. I lash out at the alarm clock, my arms flailing, until by accident more than aptitude, I hit the snooze button.

As I lie quietly in the half-dark of my room and still humid air, I can feel the emergence of a thin film of sweat. I try to drift off to sleep again, but my circadian clock is no less aware of the time than the clock on the table. I begin to notice other sounds now: the steady hum of the ice machine down the hall, and the beating of my own heart. Last night had been a blessing. Though I had not slept well, I had slept long enough to achieve something akin to a night's rest. Still, the knot of tension in my neck has not abated; worse, it has spread tendrils through my shoulders and down into my back. The ritual sadism of too-rich hotel food and the stress of working in the Gulag that is my job, have sucked the life from me. I am a corpse on a slab, bloated and ripe for dissection.

My brain feels like an old computer running on an outdated operating system. It's not uncommon, as I move from the unconscious world to the waking world, to experience a moment of confusion before all the details of my life are properly loaded into my short-term memory. Like a pilot preparing for take-off, I run through my own personal checklist. I am in a hotel room in New York City, lower Manhattan to be exact. Check. I am on the tenth—no, that was last week—the twentieth floor of a downtown hotel. Check. I am on a temporary assignment to work on a large software development project. Check. Temporary is a relative term, as it has been well over four months since I began making the three-hour Monday morning slog up the northeast corridor from my home in Virginia. Today is Tuesday, the morning of our weekly project status meeting. My heart sinks at the very thought of it. I wish I were someplace, anyplace, other than here. Double check.

I lie in bed on my back, feeling just as tired and used up as when I lay down the night before. Morning light begins filtering past the thin veil of my eyelids, forcing me to squint. An inner voice whispers faintly in my ear with the subtlety of a serpent's tongue, "Another day in the factory."

One: A Day in the Life of a Fat Man

. . . .

Just then, the clock starts its incessant buzzing again. "Get up, get up!" I roll onto my side and reach for it; then, with much effort, sit up and pivot to the edge of the bed. I slump here for a moment and wait for the room to stop spinning and the headache to subside. It takes effort to do a lot of things these days. Many feel aches and pains when they first wake up, but for me, a middle-aged man of forty-three, beset with asthma, high blood pressure and an astonishing body weight, they represent just the beginning of another twenty-four hours of humiliation and misery.

Amid grunts and audible popping sounds coming from my joints, I rise from the bed and stumble past the clothes strewn about the floor to the window. Aches and pains ricochet through my body, from my ears to my ankles and back again. I feel like I've been hit with a blast of buckshot from point-blank range, and yet, I am so accustomed to feeling this way, I hardly notice it anymore. My only concern on this late spring morning, as it has been every morning recently, is just figuring out how I will make it through another day. I part the curtains and squint into the full light of a New York morning. I'm looking south across Battery Park. The view of the Hudson River is obscured by an apartment building directly in front of me. To the left, a fortress of buildings obliterates the horizon. Here and there, I can see morning ferries and tug boats crisscrossing the grey waters of the Hudson and beyond that, a swath of the Jersey shore. Twenty floors down, West Street bustles with early morning traffic.

I have what some might call a dream job: a high-profile position on a major corporate project, company-paid expenses and one of the greatest cities in the world at my feet. And yet I can't get past the simple fact that I'm not enjoying any of it. Certainly my weight is a factor, but is it the primary factor? Before writing this book, I would have been unsure of the answer to that question, but I now know that the two hundred extra pounds I carried with me everyday were like a thick, opaque lens through which every thought and every experience of my life were filtered.

As I stand here, I wonder what Mary and the girls are doing back home in Virginia. At six o'clock in the morning, they're probably still asleep. The separation has been difficult for all of us. I should feel good, after all, because I am fulfilling the chief duty of manhood, which is to provide for one's family. As the sole breadwinner, I am doing just that. In fact, I take a certain masochistic pride in the fact that through it all, I am still holding up. But this is just testosterone-induced bravado. The fact is, I feel as though I am letting them down. By my own estimation, I have fallen far short of the goals I had set for myself as a husband and father.

My relationship with Mary has suffered because, when I get right down to it, I don't really like who I am. My weight and the associated health problems make me feel weak, a failure; it's hard to give love when you don't have any to spare for yourself. Mary has her own problems: a fifty-pound surplus of body weight and an even deeper emotional scar she has carried since childhood. The two of us are like speeding cars on a collision trajectory, our combined problems magnifying the force of impact. Worse still, I perceive that our joint failure at setting a good example is priming our daughters for a lifetime of pain and suffering.

I shower and dress quickly. I always do, because being fat means that your wardrobe is severely limited, making the decision of what to wear most mornings a no-brainer. I pull on a pair of dark pants and tuck in a white dress shirt. A light-weight tan sweater goes over the shirt. I choose the sweater even though the weather is warming up. When you're my size, sweaters tend to soften the contrast between the mound of belly fat and your lower body. On this day, I will wear a heavy leather coat over my sweater, as the evenings in New York are still quite cool.

I look in the mirror and unconsciously sneer at the man who returns my stare. My face is puffed and swollen, with the beginnings of dark circles forming around my eyes to complement the darkening splotches on my cheeks. At six feet tall, I am above average height, but the overall effect is ruined by the rolling mounds of flesh that pour down from my chest, ending abruptly in a great orbital ring of fat around my midsection. The once-youthful shimmer of my skin is gone, replaced with a flat and ashen mask, reminding me of the last glimpse of my father as he lay in his coffin.

Between my waist and my neck, I'm almost round. My clothes

always fit poorly. Sometimes they are too large, sometimes too small. I am always out of fashion. This isn't because of a lack of availability of stylish clothing. The fashion industry caters rather well to the ever-expanding waistline of the American male, but given the exorbitant prices for big-sized clothing—almost a penalty for being overweight—many simply cannot afford to buy better clothes.

I can feel swelling in my hands. My feet, with their poor circulation and blackened toenails, thankfully hidden in my shoes, look like something from a B-grade horror movie. The specter of diabetes that has shadowed three members of my immediate family haunts me daily.

The tired, dull eyes that stare back at me are hardly recognizable as my own. Although I still retain a memory of what I used to look like, I do not recognize this man in the mirror.

The circumference of my waist, being nearly equal to my height, requires me to wear my pants farther down, around my hips. I never liked wearing suspenders, because hitching my pants high up on the waist makes me look too much like the Pentecostal preachers who shepherded the churches of my youth. When I do wear a belt, the weight of my overhanging stomach rubs against the buckle, creating a painful abrasion that sometimes breaks the skin and bleeds. Some days it is so painful I have to go to the restroom at work and stuff a wad of tissue paper between my stomach and the belt buckle.

It occurs to me that life with obesity is like my belt, an ever-tightening cord that is slowly cutting me off from everything and everyone I know. Some days are worse than others, but these days, it seems there are no good days left. As bad as this morning is, it is about to get worse.

7:30 A.M.

I go down to the hotel restaurant for breakfast. I am usually still full from my evening meal and often skip breakfast, but being full and being satiated are two different things. I order from the buffet menu and have an omelet, large helping of grits,—I was amazed to find grits in New York City—orange juice and sausage. Eating in public carries with it a special risk and countless opportunities for humiliation. I try to ignore the stares, the sidelong glances and the way some people's eyes dart briefly to take in my stomach before reestablishing eye contact. The hostess is an attractive young woman who is all smiles and kind words, but I know or think I know what she and everyone else in the restaurant is thinking: look at that fat guy stuff himself with food.

8:00 A.M.

The walk to the office is difficult. It's only a few blocks, but it feels like miles to me, even though it's mostly downhill. I know I'll have to come back this way in the evening and do not look forward to it. New Yorkers have seen it all, so I'm almost relieved to discover that I don't draw as many stares as usual. I don't see many children on the street in lower Manhattan during morning rush, but on this day a mother and child about five years old rush by. The kid is wailing for something, but stops mid-wail to gawk at me. Mom glances at me for a moment then pulls him forward and the wail picks up again. I imagine he's probably begging for sweets and can hear, if only in my mind, his mother warning him that if he eats too much candy, "You'll wind up like that fat man."

Even though it is cool in the mornings, my size and poor condition cause my internal furnace to heat up quickly. By the time I get to my building several blocks away, I'm almost out of breath. I nod to the security guard as I make my way to the elevators. The lobby is nearly empty. As I step onto the elevator, my mind is preoccupied with the coming events of the day, so I am unprepared for what happens next.

One moment I'm in mid-stride with one leg raised above the threshold of the elevator. The next, when my foot comes down and touches the elevator floor, my left knee gives out. For an instant, I'm in danger of crashing to the floor, but I catch myself and stumble against the wall. This isn't the first time this has happened, but I note with a sense of disquiet that it is happening with greater frequency. Joint and mobility problems are common complaints of the morbidly obese. I wonder how long will it be before I can no longer walk without aid?

One: A Day in the Life of a Fat Man

· ·

I finally make it up to my floor where I collapse at my desk. I'm sweating profusely and breathing heavily. I wipe the sweat from my brow, but more pours out of me. The white shirt beneath the sweater I'm wearing is soaked through. It takes several minutes for my breathing and my racing heart to return to normal. It will take twenty minutes or more for my shirt to dry out. For those people who say the obese should "just get out and exercise," I have this to say: try walking in my shoes for a day.

9:00 A.M.

I work as a software design liaison between my company and an outside contractor. I spend most of my day sitting in meetings or at a desk. This is the blessing and the curse of modern technology, which makes possible enhanced productivity through the use of computers, while exacting a heavy toll on our health.

Like the animals on a modern day factory farm, I feel trapped, unable to direct the course of my own future. The vending machine down the hall spits out soda for twenty-five cents a can—such a deal. High-calorie, low-nutrient donuts, bagels, pizza and other goodies are regularly supplied by my employer. My coworkers and I often eat hurriedly at our desks, barely tasting the food. We are like beef on the hoof, fattened up on a high-grain diet and crowded into a feed lot awaiting slaughter at the whim of our corporate masters. Sometimes when I close my eyes, I can almost hear mooing.

The hours are often long, and due to the complexity of the work, problems—or should I say, "challenges," the politically correct corporate euphemism—are legion. Along with these "challenges" comes a super-sized helping of stress. I am about to get my first serving at our morning meeting. The room in which the meeting is held is ridiculously small for the number of people attending. I get there early so I can pick a seat at the table that's easy to get to and doesn't require others to squeeze past me. Other people begin streaming into the room. Everyone looks as though they've enjoyed a better night's rest than I did. They look crisp and freshly attired; I look worn and feel worse, and the day has only just begun. I try to keep up with the discussion, but find that I'm having a difficult time concentrating. This is a growing and more frequent problem. When it's my turn to report, I stumble through my script in a lifeless monotone, not sure whether I'm making any sense and hoping no one asks any questions.

10:00 A.M.

An unexpected meeting comes up that is located in another building a couple of blocks away. This is bad news because it means that not only will I have to go walking, but I won't be alone. When I'm walking by myself, I can walk at my own pace, stopping now and then to rest, but I know I'll have to keep pace with the energetic young man who will accompany me to the meeting. We start out along Broad Street and head toward the end of the block, not far from the Stock Exchange. A left turn takes us up a long incline toward Broadway. My heart is pounding. Pride prevents me from admitting that I need to rest. The leather coat makes me feel like I'm wearing a portable sauna, and my breathing is barely under control. Talking is difficult. By the time we arrive at the meeting, I am drenched and exhausted. For the next ten minutes, so much sweat pours from my head and face that I look like a fountain in a park. I certainly feel as though I weigh as much. The only thing missing, I muse, is the pigeons.

12:00 P.M.

There are problems—there always are—with the project. Another unscheduled meeting comes up. I've barely returned from my last appointment when I have to go out again, this time for a lunch meeting with one of the project's principal clients, as well as a group of managers from my company. The restaurant is close by, but small. I find that I have difficulty negotiating the narrow passages between tables to get to my seat. The shirt beneath my sweater is still damp and as I sit there, I can sense that a few buttons have come undone and that my shirttail has crept up out of my pants.

One of the problems with being obese is that when you sit at a table, your stomach forces you to sit much farther away from the table than normal. Food has to travel a greater distance from the plate to your mouth. Spills occur often. I'm careful to order the salmon as it is relatively easy to control, unlike spaghetti or a salad, which would have been a disaster. I thank God that at least we're at a table and not a booth. Booths have no equal in the amount of physical discomfort and public humiliation they offer to the obese. They are the modern-day equivalent of a medieval "iron lady," designed to force fat people to choose between talking and breathing.

Just as I'm beginning to settle into the conversation and forget about my personal troubles, disaster strikes. Because I jut so far out into the aisle, one of the waiters, balancing a tray of coffee cups and cream, bumps into me and spills cream all over my back. I can feel the cold, viscous liquid creeping down my shirt. The waiter grabs a towel and between apologies begins sopping up the cream as best he can. He implores me to remove my sweater so that he can have it cleaned at the restaurant's expense.

Everyone at my table and the tables around me is staring. I am now faced with a difficult choice: remove my sweater and reveal my sweat-stained, ill-fitting, partially unbuttoned shirt and the mounds of flesh beneath, or refuse the offer to have my sweater cleaned and look like the village idiot in front of the entire restaurant. I choose to be an idiot and lamely try to laugh off the incident, declining the waiter's offer.

I think this scene can't get any worse, but I am wrong. Now the restaurant manager, a young attractive woman, comes over and again insists that I remove my sweater so the restaurant can have it cleaned. It isn't often that strange women demand I undress in public, so I find I'm at a loss for words. I tell her I'm from out of town and she counters that she'll have the sweater sent to wherever I live. The restaurant is nearly dead silent as I struggle for a response.

"No it's OK, really," I mutter.

My table mates are looking at me now as though I really am from another world. It feels like ages before the hum of normal conversation picks up again and people return to their business. Whatever opinion my coworkers at the table had of me when we entered the restaurant,

I'm now sure it is markedly different when we leave. In a final stab of humiliation, as we're leaving the restaurant, the manager asks me once more whether I would like to have my sweater cleaned. I thank her and reply that I'm staying just a few blocks away and will go change clothes after lunch. To add a final insult to my injury, I tip the coat girl far more than she deserves. No one mentions the incident on the walk back to the office. I step across a large metal grate in the street through which the sound and the fury of a passing subway train can be heard. I find myself wishing the grate would give way and swallow me up.

2:00 P.M.

I spend the rest of the day hiding at my desk. I need a shower and feel sticky in clothes that have been twice dampened by sweat and once by cream. It's starting to rain outside.

Usually at about this time, I get drowsy and nod off. I try to stay awake by keeping busy making phone calls and attacking my to-do list. These episodes of midday sleepiness usually pass in about an hour.

3:00 P.M.

Another meeting. I have a phone call and arrive late. There's no place to sit, so I stand. My lower back is killing me. Someone leaves early and I grab his chair. Halfway into it, I discover that it's too small for me. I'm wedged between the armrests. If I try to stand up, the chair will come with me, so I squeeze into it. Everyone pretends not to notice my predicament.

4:00 P.M.

Andy, one of the guys in the office, invites me to come along to dinner with a group of programmers. I pretend to consider the offer before declining. I've learned that a dinner invitation means strolling aimlessly for blocks until the group discovers a restaurant that looks interesting. The last time I accepted a dinner invitation, the exhausting walk to the restaurant killed my appetite while the walk back, as difficult as it was on a full stomach, only made me hungry shortly after I returned to my room.

Every day I vow to accept the dinner invitations from the New York staff and accompany them to one of the many restaurants in the area. Every night I find another reason not to. The reasons typically fall into one of three categories: work, family or illness. Tonight was "illness" night. I tell them that I must be coming down with something and need to get to bed early. Andy smiles and says something about "the next time then."

There's always a next time when you're obese. The next diet will be the one that works for me, or next week I'm really going to try harder to exercise more. We spend most of our working day in hopeful yet hopeless anticipation of the next this, the next that, which never comes.

By the end of the day, I'm drenched and exhausted. At least today, I'll actually get to leave at a respectable hour. On some days, people stay here all night. The glamorous world of software development isn't so glamorous for me.

5:00 P.M.

Rain has been falling in a light, steady drizzle ever since the early afternoon, creating puddles everywhere. The evening rush of foot traffic pours out of the buildings and surges into the street. People walk with heads down, eyes forward, rushing past me as though I am a large stone in the midst of a great silent river. I lumber up a long wide alleyway that inclines toward Broadway. The hotel is still several blocks away, but it feels like I've already walked several miles. The trauma of walking uphill after a long day of meetings intensifies the pain in my lower back. It grows worse with each step. I can feel the eyes of the crowd all around me, can feel the suffocating waves of pity and disgust that threaten to drown me.

As I step off a curb, my foot sinks into a puddle of water. After months of walking through dirty snow and water, my shoes are ruined and now they are soaked through to the socks. I heave myself forward, dodging a cab before reaching the opposite curb.

5:20 P.M.

I sit on the edge of the bed in my small sterile room, my sweater lying crumpled behind me. Slumped and lifeless, I resemble a large pile of dirty laundry. The bedding is violently disturbed where I collapsed soon after arriving. The excruciating pain in my lower back and joints give me little choice. Some nights on the walk back to the hotel I barely make it to the privacy of the lobby elevator before collapsing in pain against the wall. I am tired inside and out.

6:00 P.M.

Recovered from my evening walk, I decide to order dinner in my room. I almost always eat dinner in my room. The hotel restaurant is more than adequate, but after previous visits there, where the hostess seated me so far toward the back of the restaurant I could smell the dish washing liquid in the kitchen, I took the hint. New York probably has more restaurants per square mile than any other city, but going out is just not realistic for someone like me. I shift from the bed to a tight-fitting desk chair, and absentmindedly flip through the pages of the room service menu. This is just a formality, as I have it practically memorized.

"Hello Mr. Morris, this is Paul. How may I help you tonight?"

The voice belongs to the guest services manager. It is overtly pleasant to the point of flatness. Paul and the room service staff like me. I keep them busy, tip well and am conscientious about placing the service table outside my room and phoning the desk to have someone pick it up. If the old maxim "you are what you eat," is true, Paul knows me better than he does most of the hotel's guests, as he has taken my calls many times before. Thus our familiar conversation begins.

"I'd like to order some dinner."

"Excellent Mr. Morris. Would you like to hear our special tonight?"

The line is silent for a moment. "Sure," I respond. It really doesn't matter what the special is, I've had a hard day and I need a heavy dose of comfort to put it behind me. I already know what I want.

One: A Day in the Life of a Fat Man

. . . .

"We start with a spicy tomato bisque soup followed by the main course, a fillet of mesquite grilled sea bass infused with truffle oils." As he works this culinary aria, the pitch and tenor of Paul's voice changes, rising in melodic refrain phrases. "That comes with seared asparagus spears on a bed of wild rice with fresh scallions and hand-picked mushrooms." A breathless pause follows as Paul gathers himself for the climax of this mini-opera. "For dessert, this meal includes your choice of honey-glazed baked apples in a red wine sauce or poached pears in a fragrant hibiscus-scented syrup presented in a delicate web of spun sugar."

Then I hear the abrupt sound of a breathless exhalation as Paul cools down from the exertion. I rock back in the ill-fitting chair and wait for a moment to lend the impression that I am actually considering the special.

"Uh no, I think I'd like to go with the steak tonight."

A disappointed silence follows, then having recovered, Paul replies, "Excellent. Is that the house steak or the porterhouse?"

The house steak is a dainty seven ounces of meat, while the porterhouse weighs in at over a pound of gut-busting Colorado beef, bathed in butter and herbs.

"I'll have the porterhouse."

"How would you like that?" The color has deserted Paul's voice.

"Medium well."

"That comes with a seafood chowder or garden salad. Which would you prefer?"

"Salad."

"Dressing?"

"Ranch. And could you put some chicken on that salad?"

"Of course. Would you like fries or mashed potatoes with your steak?"

"Fries."

"Something to drink?"

"A Coke."

"Would a Pepsi be OK?"

"Sure."

"Dessert?"

It goes like this for a moment more. The conversation is familiar to both of us. Like two actors with a well-rehearsed script, we speak our lines with the conviction of an opening night performance. I hang up the phone and reach for the television remote, then pause and reach for the phone instead. Dinner is a half hour away. I wheel the chair around and open the in-room snack bar and smile when I discern that the cache of Snickers candy bars has been replenished.

6:30 P.M.

A room service attendant brings dinner on a table tray. I sit in the ill-fitting desk chair and watch TV while I eat. Except for the prehistoric dinner rolls, which would need to be carbon-dated to determine their age, the food is neither good nor bad. It simply does what all my meals do, which is to fill the hole in my belly. But never, ever do my meals leave me satisfied.

8:00 P.M.

I spend the rest of the evening sprawled uncomfortably on the bed, watching TV and flipping through the pages of a magazine. Despite the bloated feeling in my stomach and the general sense of unease that always comes after eating, I eventually attack the snack bar. In a half-hearted attempt to watch my fat intake, I skip the cookies this time and choose a can of sickeningly sweet, but stale, peanuts. They taste as though they've been languishing in a warehouse since the Reagan administration.

The willingness to eat just about anything, whether we like it or not, is one of the puzzling mysteries of the overeater. In retrospect, I realize that my insatiable cravings were the result of chronic malnourishment. This is why my meals never left me satisfied.

Before bed, I take my blood pressure medication.

One: A Day in the Life of a Fat Man

....

2:00 A.M.

My eyes snap open. I sit up abruptly in bed, although with difficulty. I'm choking and there's a burning sensation in my throat. Acid? I cough violently, trying to clear my airway. It takes a moment to remember where I am. The chunk, shush, chunk of the ice machine fills in the blanks for me. I was dreaming that I drowned.

Dreams of drowning are not uncommon for obese people suffering from a life-threatening disorder known as sleep apnea. Obstructive sleep apnea, the variant from which I suffered, is a condition in which the airway at the back of the throat becomes temporarily blocked. The sufferer can experience frequent (as many as sixty per hour) moments of interrupted breathing. These episodes can persist throughout the night, inhibiting access to the kingdom of deep and restful sleep. Snoring, daytime sleepiness and an inability to concentrate are all potential consequences of sleep apnea. Heart attack, high blood pressure and stroke are also associated with this condition.

The pressure on my bladder cannot be ignored; disoriented, I fumble through the darkened room to the toilet. I don't trouble myself with the light switch, as my aim is no better in the light than it is in the dark. My habits have grown steadily more piggish. The longer I'm in New York, the worse I feel, the more I eat and the less I care. It is a familiar pattern that I recognize and fear, but I feel helpless to stop it. I exit the bathroom, stopping to retrieve a Pepsi from the snack bar, then step gingerly over the growing pile of clothes on the floor to the faint outline of the window across the room. Parting the curtains, I look out on a city not quite asleep.

In the pale light of a pastel moon, New York takes on a ghostly radiance, like a canvas in translucent hues of white. In the distance, I can see the Jersey shore, loosely sketched by rows of yellow and white lights. A lone tugboat, lit up like a Christmas tree, moves silently across the water. Below me an occasional car passes, heading south, toward the West Street terminus.

6:00 A.M.

I wake up early, squinting into the dawn light that invades the room. At some point in the night, I stumbled from my uncomfortable bed and collapsed into the uncomfortable easy chair, where I managed to sleep fitfully. The heavy meal from the previous evening leaves me dazed. I feel as though a weight greater than my own is pinning me to the chair. My mouth is parched, and thirst gnaws at me despite the evidence of several empty Pepsi cans on the desk, which I have only the faintest memory of drinking. On my first attempt to rise, my joints and unused muscles groan and protest with the effort. I fall back and contemplate what lies ahead.

Looking back, I cannot say how I managed the burden of morbid obesity for as long I did. Perhaps as my mother used to say: "It was my faith that brought me." Faith can be a wonderful thing, a powerful motivator that sees us through the dark hours when our lives seem hopeless and full of bitter discontent. But faith is a double-edged sword. Applied in the wrong way, for the wrong cause, blind faith can be an anchor that pulls us down into the murky depths of self-destruction. It was blind faith that nearly destroyed me, and continues to destroy the lives of millions.

One: A Day in the Life of a Fat Man

. . . .

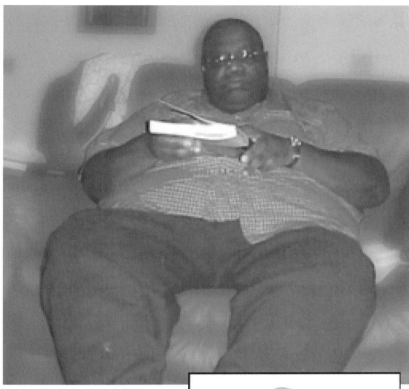

Above: Here I am just before relocating to the East Coast. Leaving our family behind in Arizona was a tough decision, but as I said to Mary, "This move will be an opportunity for us to recreate ourselves." Little did I know how true were those words.

Right: Here I am today.

Chapter Two

How Did I End Up Here?
How a fit guy like me wound up
in a fat place like this

How did this happen? How did I wind up morbidly obese and sleepless in New York City? In high school, I lifted weights. In college, I was an avid runner, clocking four to twelve miles a day. I was also a hiker who regularly trekked into Arizona's rugged outdoors, from the Grand Canyon to the badlands of the southern desert.

I often rode to college on my bicycle, taking on the thirty- four-mile round trip through rush hour traffic with the tenacity of Lance Armstrong. Once, just for kicks, I walked seventeen miles home from school, under a blistering desert sun, across simmering asphalt, just to prove to myself I could do it. Most people meeting me for the first time thought that I was an athlete, so how did this happen? I have asked myself this question a thousand times and only now have I begun to realize the answer. More important, after years of unsuccessful dieting, I have finally found a solution.

No one chooses to be fat. I didn't. This revelation may come as a surprise to some, but it's true. Every day we see overweight and obese people making decisions that seem to reflect a conscious choice to be fat. The lanes and parking lots at fast food restaurants are always busy, and we seem to be spending more time in our cars and less time walking. Snarled roads, which spread out to the distant suburbs like tentacles, keep us sitting in our cars for hours on end, while we blindly devour fast food on our way home to eat processed convenience food that is little better. We willingly sacrifice our children to corporate America by plying them with sugary treats for breakfast, lunch and dinner. A cursory glance into the overloaded carts at your favorite big-box discount store reveals a heap of chemically enhanced, nutritionally deprived convenience foods. It's easy to assume that fat people really and truly choose to be fat.

This is false logic of course, which can easily be refuted. Most people understand quite clearly that while smokers may choose to smoke, no smoker chooses to be stricken with lung cancer. No drinker chooses to suffer the horrors of liver disease. How then do we explain the self-destructive behavior of smokers, alcoholics and the obese? The mechanisms that fuel this behavior, whether addiction, genetics, human physiology run amok or simply bad behavior, are open for debate. The truth is that while many people choose to engage in injurious behavior, few will admit the consequences of that behavior.

In simple terms, smokers smoke because they enjoy the sensory experience of smoking on an emotional and physiological level. Alcoholics are little different, nor are the overweight. We all engage in behavior that gives us pleasure. The problem is that for smokers, alcoholics and overeaters, these behaviors lead to dependencies. And because of ignorance about the food we eat, we find it difficult to stop. This unhealthy behavior is driven by our unmet nutritional needs and a desire for satisfaction, not by the negative consequences of the behavior.

Immersion in this cycle of satisfaction seeking leads to clouded judgment. Hormonal influences, which are only now being discovered, add to a scenario in which rational decision making becomes nearly impossible. So it was with me. This truth—that emotional and physiological dependencies make rational behavior very difficult—lies beyond the grasp of many well-intentioned health professionals who continue to focus on a simplistic, just-say-no approach to dieting.

INDUSTRIALIZATION AND MY FAMILY
From the time my grandparents began farming over a century

ago, amazing technological leaps have revolutionized the production, manufacture and distribution of food. The advent of food additive technology and genetically modified seeds has given an additional and unprecedented level of control to the industries that produce our food. The rest of us, the so-called consumers, have not fared as well.

While it may appear to us that we have unlimited control as we choose from thousands of packaged items at the supermarket, that sense of control is largely an illusion. We see a range of exotic fruits and cheeses at upscale markets, but our food choices are actually more limited than we think. Lean turkeys with oversized mutated breasts dry out in the oven on Thanksgiving because we can no longer buy naturally raised turkeys with the requisite amount of fat. We can't buy raw milk with the cream on top anymore, or beef that hasn't been raised on a diet of hormones and antibiotics. Even something as simple as finding chicken parts with the skin still on, or chicken that hasn't been soaked in "mystery broth," requires the patience of Job and the investigative powers of Sherlock Holmes.

Most of us have little idea where our food comes from, how it is produced, and how that food interacts with our bodies. Ignorance limits our ability to make the right choices about diet and nutrition since good choices can only come with good information. Artificially produced trans fats have been in our diet for decades, but our power to choose whether or not to consume these fats was effectively taken away by a profit-motivated marketplace that failed to reveal their dangers.

The industrialization of the food supply has separated us from the origins of the food we eat, a fact reflected in the history of my family. Our story provides a cautionary tale of how we came to lose control over our food and our lives.

FOUR GENERATIONS OF FOOD

My mother's parents were rural folk who began their lives amid the cluck and clatter of chickens, the mooing of cows and the comforting noises of other barnyard residents who shared their small farm. They had a tiny patch of land in a mining camp and were little more than sharecroppers. It had been less than two-score years since the signing of the Emancipation Proclamation, but the flame of self reliance burned brightly within them and fueled their dreams for a better life than their parents had known.

Grandfather served his country as a soldier before settling down once again as a farmer and country preacher. Grandmother was an avid gardener with extensive knowledge about the medicinal properties of the native plants that grew wild in the hills and hollows of rural Alabama.

When I was a child, my mother often recalled the work of hog killing, which usually began on a cold autumn morning. It was Grandfather's job to do the actual killing, a most solemn act. When that deed was done, the hog was suspended above a wood-fired cauldron filled with boiling water drawn from the well. The animal was scalded in the water and its bristles scraped clean with a dull knife. Then the hog was slit open, disemboweled, and cut into pieces. Nothing was wasted. They made head cheese from the head, rendered lard from the skin and fat and made sausage from the innards. The pork belly and ham were salted and consigned to the smokehouse. Later, some of the lard would be used to make lye soap.

My mother's parents were not rich people, and so they relied mostly on the land for their subsistence. What could not be raised, hunted, caught on a hook, grown in the garden or bartered with neighbors, was purchased from the local store. Both my mother's parents were strong and tall, judging by the stories passed down to me and the one faded photograph I have of them.

My father's parents were also farmers, resourceful and self-sufficient. Once my father took my older sister, Carol, to visit his parents on their farm in Alabama. One day, Grandmother brought in a fresh batch of eggs from the henhouse and prepared to make breakfast. A city girl, Carol protested against eating "funny tasting" eggs that had been lying on the ground only a few minutes earlier. She pleaded instead for the familiar taste of commercial eggs, trussed up in a pretty carton, which she knew could be found at the local store. Grandmother took pity on her poor misguided granddaughter, though she must have wondered what kind of children our father was raising. She dispatched a cousin to the store to buy eggs. Our cousin returned a short time later with store-bought eggs which Carol found more to her liking. What Carol didn't find out until much later, when she was nearly grown, was that those store-bought eggs had actually been sold to the local grocer by my grandmother. They had come from the very same chickens. Because they had been languishing in the store for some time, they were not as fresh as the eggs grandmother had gathered for breakfast, which accounted for the difference in taste.

My own parents were born during a transitional period in the early 1900s. They were less inclined to live the lives of their farming parents, and sought instead to follow the bright star that lay in the northern sky, seeking their fortune somewhere beyond the rural south. They lived halfway between the old world of self-reliance that belonged to their parents and the new world of dependence on automation and commercially prepared food that was the hallmark of the new century. They settled in Detroit, and lived in a succession of houses situated on small plots of land. They kept no animals, save a few cats and a dog, but in a gesture to the lifestyle they once knew, they regularly purchased live fowl from the farmers market.

My father would bring a flapping, squawking chicken home on Sundays and my older brother and sister would gather round to watch him wring the bird's neck with the deft expertise of an executioner. Despite his longing for life in the city, he could not wring the farming spirit from his soul as easily as he wrung life from the chicken.

After the chicken was scalded in hot water, my brother and sister removed the feathers. My mother would gut the chicken, cut it up into pieces for the day's meal, and save the head, feet and other miscellaneous parts to make soup. Everything was used, save the feathers and the cluck.

Without land to call their own, my parents were rootless; they journeyed to the West Coast and back again, their lives a reflection of the restlessness of the country at large. More people were moving off the land, sometimes involuntarily, to the more transient life found in America's industrial centers. Newly built highways and affordable automobiles made it difficult for anyone to stay in one place for very long. While most meals were still home-cooked, the raw ingredients for those meals increasingly came from the neighborhood store. Like so many of their generation, my parents consumed a greater share of these store-bought foods than their parents had done, and their diets included a greater percentage of refined flour and sugar. The result was the onset of excess weight and obesity in their middle years. Clearly this change was not due to a lack of exercise, as my father was a construction laborer who knew the meaning of a hard day's work. My mother did everything from backbreaking domestic work to harvesting produce beneath a sweltering sun.

MY MOTHER'S KITCHEN

There was a time when no one in my family thought about dieting. Although some family members carried excess weight, dieting and the associated fear of food were uncommon. Food had a special meaning in our lives: more than just fuel, and more than just nourishment, food occupied a place as vital as our faith and our love for each other. Even until the 1970s, the preparation and consumption of food remained a fundamental part of the traditions and rituals that bound us together.

While our neighbors' houses might have differed in size and quality of furnishings, the kitchen was the common denominator in every home. The refrigerators, stoves and sinks in the homes of my friends and extended family were all pretty much the same. The mouth-watering vision of a rib roast, the intoxicating aroma of homemade cookies, or the snap of green peas fresh from the garden were familiar sensory experiences, providing us all with a sense of kinship.

My mother's kitchen would never have made the cover of a designer magazine, although it was the most important room in our little house with its peach-colored stucco exterior and dark green trim. The house was built shotgun style, which meant you could stand at the open front door and look down the length of the house through the kitchen and out the open back door.

The place where Mama prepared our family meals was a narrow

room with a creaky tile floor and a pale green ceiling darkened with cooking smoke. It was a tunnel of delightful smells and tastes that joined our living room, in the front of the house, to an enclosed porch at the rear. Mama cooked on an old gas stove that was like a fire-breathing dragon. More than once, while trying to light the pilot, each of us (we were five children) had been surprised by a frightening belch of blue flame that singed our eyebrows and filled us with fear.

The counter top between the stove and refrigerator was covered with pink Formica, which had a playful 1950s pattern vaguely reminiscent of atoms. It held a double sink of chipped porcelain. We called the refrigerator an ice box even though none of us kids had ever seen a real ice box. That term, like so many other orphaned words from my mother's generation, had yet to disappear from our collective unconscious.

Opposite the working side of the kitchen was a large horizontal freezer which, in times of plenty, we kept stocked with cuts of beef, numerous chickens, a turkey or two, pork from the squeal to the tail and fresh fish purchased at the grocery store or, when we were lucky, received as a gift from our neighbor, drawn from the depths of the desert lakes that lie in the northern mountains. Low-fat dieting, calorie counting and carb-watching were not part of our lexicon or that of anyone else we knew.

A small square table with thin metal legs, shaky and insecure, stood beside the freezer. I often sat there in the evening hours, after the family meal, diligently doing homework.

My mother used heavy stainless steel pots and black-iron skillets to cook up collard greens and chili beans, scramble eggs and country-fry chicken. Soups and broths simmered patiently for hours and filled our home with delectable smells.

On cold mornings, we ate steaming bowls of oatmeal with raisins and cream, buttered grits with cheese, or flapjacks stacked three high and smothered in butter, with sticky sweet, homemade syrup. Cornbread and homemade rolls awaited that first kiss of sweet butter when they came from the oven—a memory that still makes me smile from the inside out. We bought log-sized loaves of longhorn cheese from the grocer and sometimes fresh eggs from our neighbors, whose errant rooster I often pursued whenever he wandered away from his flock. Our milkman delivered full-fat cow's milk and goat's milk, in thick glass bottles, fresh from the dairy.

No, my mother's kitchen would never have made the cover of a designer magazine, but it will remain for me the paradigm of what a kitchen should be. Today, our modern kitchens are as big as living rooms and fitted with islands, Italian tile and massive steel ovens. We spend thousands for top-of-the-line cookware, custom countertops and the latest appliances. We tune in to the Food Channel on cable TV and marvel at the incredible creations of our favorite chefs. We collect cookbooks that cater to every conceivable taste and style of cuisine.

And what do we do with all this technology and potential? We order pizza. And on those rare occasions when we really want to "do something special" for our loved ones, we open a can, box or bag with a list of ingredients we can neither pronounce nor comprehend and nuke the damnable contents in the microwave. This is the state of "cooking" in the twenty-first century. What happened?

THE GARDEN OF EARTHLY DELIGHTS
Spring in Phoenix, Arizona always came quietly to Jefferson Street. The change of seasons in the desert valley was subtle but inescapable. The bristly saguaro in front of Reddy's Corner store would display its snow white blossoms while tentacles of Bermuda grass spread out to reclaim barren patches of dirt in the lawn. Our front yard was a butterfly's haven in spring, with its fist-sized zinnia blossoms, fragrant roses and soft white oleander petals.

While we got much of our food from the grocery store, we also supplemented our diet with wild catfish and trout, farm-raised chickens, wild rabbit and even deer meat. But of all the ways the working-class neighbors of Jefferson Street stretched their meager paychecks, gardening was the favorite.

Gardening in the desert was both a blessing and a curse. The temperate weather meant that you could grow food nearly year-round, but the desert clay was hard and unforgiving. The neighborhood I grew up in was populated by poor people. Few, if any, had anything beyond a high school education. They were all pioneers of the great Diaspora, Africa's children wandering in the wilderness of America. Only two generations removed from slavery, they discovered that life in the North was no easier than it had been in the South, so they migrated west, still in search of their own promised land. They were Americans in the purest sense of the word, possessed of a strong work ethic and enough optimism to believe in the messages of pride and self-determination that were delivered in the hand-me-down sermons of Frederick Douglass and Booker T. Washington. That sense of pride and practicality found expression in the backyard vegetable gardens of nearly every home on the block, testaments to a deep desire for self-reliance.

My mother was a master gardener, the neighborhood's Demeter, coaxing green life from the barren Sonoran desert clay. She was a tall woman, heavy-set, with a stern face and broad shoulders. Her hair was almost straight, jet black streaked with grey. She loved working outdoors, although I thought she loved watching me and my brother David working more. Mother was from Alabama, a place where the whole world was green. It was there, from her mother, that she learned to garden. In Arizona, she grew tall stalks of sweet yellow corn, impatient for melted butter and the company of a tender rack of ribs. Deep green collards, honeyed melons and sweet ripe tomatoes, too delicious to wash before eating, provided a rich return on the difficult investment of gardening in desert clay. Grapefruits, tangerines and oranges practically grew wild in our backyard. Our garden always produced more than we could eat and so we shared our bounty with friends, family and even strangers.

It was in the garden that I learned the rewards of hard work and saw first hand the connection between the land and myself. To use pesticides in our garden was unthinkable. The garden taught me the art of patience as I waited for the warm days of summer and the sweet melons that came with the season. The garden taught me the importance of responsibility when it was my job to keep our dogs out, and the price of irresponsibility when I didn't. When our crop of grapes failed to thrive, even after all our hard work digging, planting and nurturing, I learned that failure and loss are part of living and that we can only do our best, learn from our mistakes and move on.

I wish I could say that I carried these lessons with me all my life, but like many of us, I forgot or discarded many of them. But a lesson once learned can be relearned and reapplied to one's life. Good food, self-reliance and a love for community, these were the treasures nurtured to fruition by the residents of Jefferson Street. This, their promised land, was a garden of earthly delights.

THE WINDS OF CHANGE

Although my mother was skilled in the growing arts, as time progressed, the food she put on the table reflected the transition we all experienced, from home-grown, home-cooked foods to prepared commercial food.

In the late 1960s, we found ourselves in economic peril. My father disappeared from our lives one day and never came back. He had taken these breaks from the rigors of domestic responsibility before and always returned, but this time we would not see him again until his death. Saddled with the responsibility of five children, my mother went to work. She had training as a nurse's assistant, but in those less enlightened days, she could not find such work in Arizona and so became a domestic servant instead.

We stretched our meager income with food from the government "Commodity Program." Every few weeks, we received a ration of food that included canned spam for meat, powdered milk in a big white box, bottles of clear corn syrup, peanut butter, canned vegetables and dry goods like white flour, rice and pinto beans. The program was correctly named—these were commodities! On rare occasions we got cheese.

The corner convenience store a block away from my home was a trove of candy bars and soda pop. We were too poor to afford either on a regular basis, but when we did indulge in these empty foods, it was a "special treat."

At school, the breakfast and lunchtime menus included cold cereals, waffles, milk, burgers, fries, lasagna and drippy sloppy Joe sandwiches. There's no doubt that the commodity and school lunch programs saw my family through some tough times, but the inescapable fact was that these foods were heavily weighted toward refined carbohydrates, the very foods now blamed for the obesity epidemic.

At home, my family's diet slowly changed from mostly whole foods to the newer convenience foods. Store-bought bread that turned to paste in your mouth replaced home-baked bread. TV dinners were cheap and easy to prepare. Adulterated foods that were either deficient in fat or comprised of poor quality fats slowly replaced our dietary staples. Powdered milk, margarine and vegetable shortening were less expensive, more convenient and supposedly healthier than whole milk, butter and lard. We switched to so-called healthy polyunsaturated vegetable oils which we would discover, years later, were highly susceptible to rancidity, making them harmful to the body. Hot oatmeal with butter and whole milk gave way to cold cereals that were nutritionally suspect and packed a wallop of extra carbohydrates and calories. Sugared drinks slowly began to replace milk.

Though not fat, I was a big kid in grade school; but I feared I would grow fat in time, so in high school I became obsessed with fitness and managed my weight through relentless exercise. In college I had less time to work out and the weight gain began. Not much at first, as I still managed to find time to engage in marathon sessions of exercise, but I noticed that despite my efforts, I was beginning to lose ground in my battle to stay trim. By the time I graduated from college and entered the world of work on a full-time basis, my processed food diet and the nine-to-five grind conspired to escalate my weight gain dramatically. I didn't realize it at the time, but my struggle with weight gain had begun at a younger age for me than for my parents. My grandparents never had a problem with excess weight.

By the time my own generation came of age, the days of live

and barnyard smokehouses had faded from memory. The first house Mary and I bought, in Phoenix, and the land upon which it sat, were even smaller than my parent's, but cost several times more. Meat came wrapped in plastic from the grocery store freezer, subject to the yellow glow of artificial lights. Half my meals were eaten outside the home and many of those that were consumed at home came pre-cooked, to be thawed and reheated in a microwave. The food I ate came with a cargo of additives, extenders, flavorings and enhancers that didn't even exist in my grandparents' time.

I didn't know and didn't care where my food came from, how it was produced and whether or not the additives were good for me. All I did care about was taste and the fact that it was it cheap. By the time I reached adulthoood, the only remaining dietary connection between me and my grandparents was gardening.

By the 1990s, America had completely bought into the shaky logic of the diet-heart hypothesis, which labeled dietary fat and cholesterol as the primary causes of heart disease. We went lowfat—at least we thought we did. What we didn't realize was that we had replaced the healthy traditional fats in our diet with processed vegetable oils and trans fats while gradually increasing our intake of refined carbohydrate foods—sugars and starches. Parallel advances in technology made our lives physically easier as our cities emptied themselves in a mass migration to the suburbs. We were becoming a nation of sedentary people, spending more time in our cars on the commute to the "burbs" while eating more high-calorie, nutrient-poor foods that rarely satisfied and only left us wanting more.

By the time I became a father in 1990, I was completely sold on the lowfat, high-carb, convenience food craze. I ate tofu, joined a gym, dieted religiously, became a vegetarian, and still packed on the weight on my way to over four hundred pounds. My first daughter followed in my footsteps at an earlier age, gaining weight at an alarming rate after the age of eight.

In our house we had a kitchen, but what usually went on there could hardly be described as cooking. Most of our meals came out of a box, bag or can, or they came by way of a pimply-faced kid delivering pizza. Though Mary was gaining weight at a slower pace than I was, she had filled out considerably and no longer resembled the woman I married.

We knew that the problem was with our diet, so we vowed again and again to eat less, cut the fat and exercise more. . . .but none of this worked. When my second daughter began to get fat at the age of seven, Mary and I cursed ourselves for not setting a better example, but how could we? We couldn't help ourselves.

Beginning in the late 1900s through the latter half of the twentieth century, two generations of my family lived and died. From our family history, a pattern emerged. As each generation surrendered more and more of its independence to an increasingly industrialized food supply and the corporate kitchen, the less healthy that generation became. As processed convenience foods with their additives and their extended shelf life became the primary source of sustenance for my family, I saw a corresponding increase in weight gain and obesity. Medical problems, from asthma to diabetes, sleep apnea and obesity, were occurring sooner with each succeeding generation.

Despite the progress made in food production, and despite America's miraculous ability to feed the world, in one small corner of that world my family was losing ground. We were more dependent on strangers to feed us, saw our youth interrupted with illness sooner, and were dying at an earlier age.

My parents had been trim and healthy well into their thirties, only succumbing to weight problems later in life. When I was young, two of my four siblings were already overweight, born, apparently, with a "genetic" tendency toward excessive weight. In my own family, both of my children and my wife were overweight, and I was obese. Yet my grandparents were trim all their lives. What was happening to us? It was as though a family curse had been lain upon us, growing worse with each succeeding generation.

On those long nights in New York when I sat alone in my room, I thought a lot about my family. Dietary chaos reigned on the home front.

I felt helpless to do anything about it. What was to become of us? My children were experiencing problems with their health much earlier than I had. Would their lives become a burden for them as well?

Chapter Three

Chaos on
the Home Front
There's no place like home. . . for gaining weight

It was six o'clock in the morning on an overcast day in May of 2003. The corridor that snakes along the east coast connecting the cities of Boston, New York and Washington D.C., was already alive with commuter traffic. Interstate 95 and the Amtrak rail lines that span the corridor were already humming like living arteries, sending thousands of morning travelers to points north and south. In one of the outlying suburbs of D.C., my wife, Mary, awoke. Before she could draw her first conscious breath, the feeling that heralds unwelcome news cast a shadow over her day before it had even begun. Our conversation before I left for New York a few hours earlier was the last thing on her mind when she slipped into a restless sleep. It was the first thought to greet her when she awoke.

At three o'clock in the morning. We had been sitting together quietly, waiting in the darkened living room for a cab to take me to the train station. I was slumped on the sofa, facing a large window that looked out onto a deserted street. On these early mornings, our conversations were usually punctuated with intermittent spells of silence. After nearly seventeen years of marriage, two children, and an accumulation of over two hundred fifty pounds of unwanted body fat between us, we often found there was little to talk about. Lately, these early morning conversations had grown more solemn in tone and seemed to bring the darkness from the outside into our home and into our lives.

"I don't know how much longer I can do this," I said after a long pause.

"Do what?"

"These trips. The job. I just don't know how much longer. . . ." My voice trailed off and faded into the background noises of the house. For a time, the only sounds we could hear were the hum of the refrigerator and my labored breathing.

"Do you have everything, your tickets, your wallet?" Mary was trying to be helpful. She often took this tack when there was a truth she didn't want to face.

"I pick up my ticket at the station," I replied in a lifeless voice. There was another pause. "You need to start thinking about what you're gonna do. . . . when I'm gone."

"What do you mean? You mean today?" She was leaning forward now, but still wasn't taking the bait.

I laughed softly, but there was no joy in my voice. "I mean when I'm gone, gone."

She looked directly at me then. "Richard, what's wrong? Are you OK?"

I inhaled deeply, then coughed as the cool air hit the mucus lying in ambush somewhere along the path to my tired lungs. Another cold had found a home in my worn-out body. I told her about how difficult things had been in New York, told her about the painful days followed by the sleepless nights, told her, finally, about the sense of hopelessness that was slowly drowning me.

"I feel used up, tired. I just don't know how much longer I can do this." I choose my next words carefully. "I. . . . feel like I might not be around much longer."

"What. . . ." But she was interrupted by the headlights of the cab piercing the window as it turned into our driveway.

I stood up with a grunt and grabbed my travel case. "I'll call you when I get to New York," I said, then kissed her and stepped out into the dark.

As the tail lights of the cab blinked and then disappeared down the street, Mary began to cry.

Mary was a preacher's daughter. We met in college when I attended her father's church. She had plans to become a doctor. I had seen her before, at the university, usually at the library or the college of science. More than once, I considered approaching her, but I could not tell whether her purposeful stride and serious demeanor were simply the result of a focus on her destination or the outward signs of someone disinterested in consorting with a jock. I wasn't an athlete in the literal sense, but the hours of long distance running, weight-lifting and basketball made me look like one.

Mary was different then, too. Despite her modest taste in clothing, which usually bordered on drabness, she was altogether transformed in church, wearing hand-sewn dresses that revealed the supple curves and the muscular sensuousness of a beautiful young woman.

Seventeen years of marriage, two children and an incalculable number of chocolate chip cookies later, she had gained well over fifty pounds. But more than the weight that burdened her body was the burden of a life that had not turned out as expected. She had been molested at the age of twelve and left with an emotional wound that had never healed. The crime left her trapped in a dark corner of fear and self-doubt, feelings that manifested themselves in bouts of emotional darkness, thoughts of suicide and destructive overeating. Our marriage was a series of fights, a scorched earth dotted with frequent brush fires that we could never seem to extinguish for good. They were fueled by Mary's depression and triggered by my quick temper. More often than not, we doused the flames with food. Food could make you believe you were happy, at least for a short time. Now, medicated on antidepressants, Mary was coping reasonably well emotionally. For several years, life had been better, but the ground she had gained in emotional stability was quickly lost with the decline in our physical health.

A Life Unburdened

. . . .

MARY'S STORY

In Steinbeck's *The Grapes of Wrath*, the Joad family pulls up stakes and departs Depression-era Oklahoma in search of greener pastures to the west. Mary's mother grew up in the Midwest. Long after the winds of the Great Plains had swept away the dust and dreams of the "Okies," she pulled up her deeply rooted life and went in search of her own green fields. She had fire under her feet and longed to see that part of the world that lay beyond the confining borders of Eufala, Oklahoma.

Unlike her mother, Mary was born and raised in Arizona, and she expected to live there until the end of her days. When I came home one day and told her that my job was moving to the East Coast, she didn't hesitate, having decided that, like her mother, it was time to see a little bit more of the world. With children in tow, we set out for a new life.

That new life was interrupted with a six-month separation while I worked in New York. Mary had been steadily gaining weight for years. In Arizona, she worked as a respiratory therapist and later as a polysomnographer. Both jobs kept her busy and sleep-deprived, leaving precious little time for preparing nutritious meals. After we moved, Mary threw herself into a new life as a full time home-worker. Mary wore many hats—she was a mother, home school teacher, wife, bill juggler, lawn mower, chauffeur, pizza order specialist, food microwaver, and a woman who cried in the dark after the children had been put to bed. Cut loose from the support system she had known all her life, she found herself adrift in a world of indifference. She wondered daily how she would cope.

With all the changes and added pressure of her new East Coast life, Mary soon found herself tilting the scale at one hundred ninety-three pounds. Her doctor tried to be conciliatory, but Mary could sense his deep concern for her health. She was further troubled by the fact that words like "hypertension," "medication" and "obesity" had begun creeping into their conversations, words she thought would never apply to her.

As Mary's weight gain continued, her health steadily declined. She used to love hiking the rugged desert mountains of central Arizona but found herself spending more and more time hiking to the refrigerator and the grocery store. She was well on her way to becoming a not-so-proud member of the two hundred-plus club. She was wearing a size eighteen and one-half dress and knew it was only a matter of time before the question, "Do you have that in a size twenty?" would apply to her.

Moving cross-country from Arizona and the comfortable world of friends and family she had known since childhood to the unfamiliar world that was the East Coast added a layer of stress to her life that only made her physical problems worse. Now, despite the medication for her depression, the old feelings of hopelessness and despair had returned.

THE NEXT GENERATION

The sense of dread had not diminished when Raven, our younger daughter, came sleepy-eyed into the room. She climbed into bed and nudged her mother aside. With an impish gleam in her eye, she slipped beneath the covers and settled into the warm spot where Mary had been. This was part of the morning ritual, but it had taken on a new meaning in my absence. Now, a subtle sense of fear seemed to permeate everything. Raven's forays into our bed were a reflection of that fear and the uncertainty she felt at the disruption in our lives with my forced departure for New York. Equally troubling for us were the visual signs of our poor diet reflected in her. Despite her manic energy, at the tender age of eight she was gaining weight fast, already starting to thicken around the middle with a miniature alcohol-free version of a middle-aged beer gut. Worse, she was starting to show signs of the same volatile mood swings that afflicted Mary.

As for Stephanie, our older daughter, at thirteen she was nearly six feet tall. She too was overweight, slow and ponderous for her age. Her complaints of bodily aches and pains were typical of someone much older.

When Stephanie was seven years old, she was diagnosed with precocious puberty, a condition that signals the early onset of physical and hormonal development. The treatment recommended by our doctor involved a monthly hormone injection at the doctor's office. During our visits to the office, I saw the fear in her eyes and held her trembling hand as the needle bit deep into muscle, sending synthetic hormones coursing through her body. These painful injections, designed to slow her body's race to adulthood, left us in a haze of anxiety, fear and doubt. We had questions, but when my wife and I asked about the connection between early puberty and our diet, we felt the sting of the doctor's dismissive response. Eventually, we stopped the treatments—against our doctor's recommendation. No one seemed to know what causes early puberty, but it has now become so common that some members of the medical community consider the onset of puberty at the age of seven to be "normal."

Six years later, we wonder still whether we made the right decision in subjecting her to the treatment. In light of what we now know about the drug she was given and about food, particularly soy foods and their estrogenic properties that can trigger early puberty, we suspect the decision we made was wrong.

In May of 2003, we were a family sinking in a quicksand of health problems. The list of ailments that afflicted us read like a Who's Who of contemporary disorders: asthma, depression, high blood pressure, poor blood circulation, joint pain, teeth problems, headaches, poor concentration, low energy, insomnia, sleep apnea, acid reflux and poor digestion. Through it all, we dutifully took our medications and stoically accepted our various afflictions. At the center of these problems was excess weight. As our midsections expanded, so too did the number and complexity of the related illnesses, but this burden of declining health was normal, wasn't it? These things happened to everyone, didn't they?

It wasn't as though we weren't trying to find a solution. In fact, we collected diets the way Tiger Woods collected golf championships. But our scores were considerably higher. In dieting—as in golf—that's a bad thing.

Chapter Four

Dieting in the Dark
An endless search for the perfect diet
leads to places better left alone

When I was in grade school, I developed a keen interest in Greek mythology. One of the most sympathetic characters was Sisyphus. Poor Sisyphus, once employed as King of Corinth, fell on hard times after Zeus, the CEO of Greek mythology, was caught engaging in corporate misbehavior. Overcome by a sense of civic duty, Sisyphus informed on his boss. Unfortunately, ancient Greece had no whistle blower protection laws, so he was sent to Tartarus, the sub-basement of hell. There he was sentenced to roll a large boulder up a steep hill, but just before he could crest the hill, his strength would fail him and both he and the stone would tumble back down to the bottom. Sisyphus would pick himself up and begin the effort all over again. Since parole was not an option in Tartarus, Sisyphus was condemned to this back-breaking labor for all eternity.

Whenever I started a new diet, I always thought of Sisyphus. The predictable cycle of dieting—success followed by failure—made it easy to identify with his tragic story. When I compared the difficulties of weight loss to boulder rolling, I sometimes wondered whether Sisyphus had the easier of the two tasks.

It wasn't as though Mary and I had not tried to lose weight. Between the two of us, we had set off on dozens of dietary expeditions, usually some variation of the lowfat regimen that most experts recommend. Invariably these diets began with the joy of first-week weight loss but ended in the

47

sorrow of last-week weight gain. Between the hopes and disappointments, we experienced a few small victories, but those victories, in every case, were short-lived. Long-term failure was the overriding theme and the inevitable outcome of all our efforts.

Much has been written about those of us who are overweight and obese. More often than not, we are cast as the villains in life's play. We are the gluttons and idle sinners for whom the selfish quest for pleasure trumps all other concerns. Because we have chosen indulgence, we are judged worthy of scorn and justly sentenced to a life burdened by illness. Of course, most overweight people are neither gluttons nor selfish nor sinners. We do, in fact, share one virtuous trait: the unshakable faith that the next diet, the next food fad or the next medical miracle will answer our prayers.

We follow the guidelines set forth by our doctors, the diet gurus, and Aunt Esther, who lost ten pounds in two weeks on the tuna-fish-and-avocado diet, but somehow we never get the results we expect. Clearly there is a disconnect between what is believed about weight loss and what is really true. Until we discover what these truths are, we will forever be dieting in the dark. And so it was with this blind, dogged faith that Mary and I began our own tour of duty in the war against weight.

WEIGHT WATCHERS

One of the first diets I tried was Weight Watchers. I paid my dues and faithfully attended the weekly meetings. At home, I weighed my food and choked down meals that never quite satisfied my hunger, leaving me in a perpetual state of longing. Still, I had high hopes for this diet. Members met weekly to exchange ideas and encourage each other. The cell I belonged to met regularly in an unassuming strip mall. As an added benefit, I rode my bike the two miles or so to the small storefront office that served as our gathering place. The membership was overwhelmingly female, except for myself and one other man. I don't recall much of what happened in the meetings beyond the fact that they felt very much like what I imagined a support group would be like, only more upbeat. We had public weigh-ins, which were only slightly less traumatizing than public executions. There were lively discussions on food, tear-soaked announcements of weight loss or weight gain, and spirited transactions in low-fat recipes rivaling anything you might see on the trading floor of the New York Stock Exchange.

While all this was going on, the other man and I sat glumly in the back of the room and inspected our wristwatches. We attempted to talk sports and engage in other y-chromosome conversation. In the end, I grew tired of the recipe exchanges and encouragement intended to improve the taste of the low-fat diets we were all sentenced to. If these communal gatherings were necessary for success, I saw failure in my future, as I could not see myself at fifty years of age, sitting forlornly in a folding chair between two women swapping sugarless, chocolate-free, lowfat brownie recipes. I finally made the decision to "go over the wall" when my "cellmate" failed to show up one night. Perhaps if there had been a men's Weight Watchers, I would have lasted longer, but given the typical male distaste for discussions that touch on personal shortcomings, like a beer gut the size of a VW, I cannot imagine what we would have done to fill the time. I don't recall whether I lost any weight while on Weight Watchers, but I did get plenty of exercise riding my bike.

SHAKE, SHAKE, SHAKE

I saw the Slimfast commercials on TV and the ads in the magazines. Here was a weight-loss strategy that did not require attending meetings or participating in public weigh-ins. Slimfast was a powdered meal replacement drink that came in three enticing flavors—vanilla, strawberry, and chocolate. I developed a liking for strawberry and usually had one for breakfast. At first, Mary joined me in my new ritual of slurping down breakfast shakes, but in no time she abandoned the faith and left me on my own.

At first, I did lose a few pounds, and although the taste was a far cry from a real strawberry shake, it was not unpleasant. But I soon found that the satiating effect of the shakes was short-lived. It was not uncommon to drink one and still be hungry. After a time, it became more and more difficult for me to get by on just a shake as a replacement for a meal. Finally, I just stopped drinking them one day. The partially-consumed containers remained in my cupboard for months afterward, a reminder of my most recent failure.

THE INFAMOUS CABBAGE DIET

After some initial experimentation, even I knew better than to pursue this one, but the diet had come recommended to Mary by one of her sisters, and so she decided to give it a try. I remember thinking that the diet was remarkably similar to the experience of starving Europeans during World War II. Mary did not share my passion for history, so she persevered.

To be effective, the diet relied on the prodigious consumption of cabbage as the active weight-loss agent. Adherents were allowed one pitifully small hamburger patty for dinner but all other meals had to consist of cabbage, usually in the form of soup. Mary managed to stick with it for almost two weeks, but eventually succumbed to her body's craving for something more substantial. She was quickly reunited with the few pounds she had shed. Those pounds brought along some friends from wherever excess pounds go when you lose them temporarily.

THAR SHE BLOWS

The cabbage diet was followed by the tea diet, which was based on an exotic blend of tea containing as its active ingredient a powerful bowel stimulant. The predictable result was akin to launching a nuclear strike against one's colon. This diet had come recommended by yet another of Mary's sisters. Having observed the deleterious effect of the cabbage diet on Mary, I wisely abstained from further participation in unsanctioned human experiments. Mary, ever the explorer, was not dissuaded, and chose to boldly go where no right-thinking person had gone before. Mostly though, she went to the bathroom. The tea left her horribly dehydrated and afraid to eat. The prospect of another Vesuvius-like eruption from her lower regions brought a quick and merciful end to the tea diet.

Mary was one of twelve children and had an inexhaustible supply of sisters. If each one of them had a favorite diet to recommend, I feared for Mary's safety, as there was no telling how much longer she could survive their advice.

THE GYM RAT DIET

While I now knew enough to avoid any diet recommended from members of Mary's family, I was not deterred from the suggestions of "experts." I decided to follow the guidance of those diet industry gurus who insisted I was fat because I was lazy and didn't get enough exercise. This flaw in my character could easily be remedied, I reasoned, by joining a gym. I signed up with a gym less than half a mile from my home, and haunted the place day and night.

Early mornings were not so bad as the gym was usually empty and I could exercise on the better machines without interference. Evenings were another story. The happy hour crowd was an eclectic mix of lurkers, stalkers, lycra models and ladies' men who labored under the mistaken belief that a sweaty fat guy in a jogging suit was somehow irresistibly attractive to well-toned, cellulite-free spandex queens. Taking a cue from Shakespeare, I regarded the whole scene as a grand play—which I took in from my perch atop the stair machine. Often though, I had to wait in line to get a machine and invariably it was my fate to follow the sweatiest man in America, a rolling designation assigned to whoever happened to be on the treadmill or stepper ahead of me.

I was exercising two to three hours a day, putting in punishing hours on the stair climber and the weight machines. The weight fell off so fast that at one point, my gym counselor remarked that I was disappearing before her eyes. This should have been cause for celebration. I was looking like my old self again, but in fact, I was dying inside. The endless hours of exercise were wearing me down. I was bored and tired of living at the gym. I felt as though I had been sentenced to a life of hard labor. If this is what it took to lose weight, I wanted no part of it. Each time I dragged myself onto one of the many medieval instruments of torture, it was a little bit harder than the last time. I was running on the fumes of will power. Eventually, I gave up. . . and promptly regained all the weight I lost, plus—you may have guessed this already—a little bit more.

BETTER WEIGHT LOSS THROUGH SCIENCE

Despite my repeated failures at losing weight, I was not quite ready to give up completely. I had an abundance of faith in science and reasoned that if I could not accomplish this task myself, science certainly could. A visit to my doctor was arranged. With the best of intentions, he prescribed a drug, the name of which I no longer remember, but I do recall that the method of operation was reasonably straightforward. Put simply, the drug reduced the ability of my body to metabolize fat. If I consumed more fat than my body could handle—and here the doctor leaned in close, I think he enjoyed imparting this bit of news—the result would be flatulently dramatic and carry unfavorable social consequences. I considered these words for a moment, then concluded that the risk was no less socially acceptable than waddling about with a hundred pounds of excess weight. I was thus undeterred at the prospect of becoming a social pariah and eagerly took the free samples the doctor provided.

I had great expectations for this drug which had as its active ingredient what I came to refer to as "Factor F." To the dismay of a few unlucky associates, the drug worked—initially. In a very short period of time, my body responded to this new chemical assault by overriding the fat-metabolizing limits of the drug and suppressing the flatulence-generating Factor F. In no time, I was popping the pills like jellybeans. Their potency, sufficiently reduced, had little effect on my body. I did not refill the prescription.

THE RABBIT DIET

I wish I could say that the rabbit diet consisted of variations of cooked rabbit, but that was not the case. Of all the diets we attempted, the most ambitious and initially most promising was our foray into the realm of vegetarianism. I came to vegetarianism with the faith and zeal of a freshly converted sinner. In the beginning, things were great. I felt better than I had in years. I was losing weight and in my own humble opinion, looking great. But the transition was not without its challenges. While I no longer ate meat, I still had a taste for it, a disturbingly strong compulsion that rapidly consumed my every waking thought. And so it was that soy, the miraculous chameleon of foodstuffs, came to my rescue. Having frequented an Indian restaurant that catered to vegetarians, I came to love this pallid lump of flavorless vegetable matter which, with a little imagination—OK, a lot of imagination—somehow made me believe I was still eating meat. I discovered that, like a politician trolling for votes, soy could be anything you wanted it to be.

At the time, the selection of soy-based faux-meat dishes was small, and they could only be obtained for a princely sum at a local upscale grocer, the kind that catered to the Jaguar-and-brie set. At least once a week, I pulled my battered Toyota pickup with the rattling tail-gate up alongside the shining Porsches and BMWs in the parking lot and took my place in the checkout line amidst the affluent class. At least I could truly boast to my fellow health-conscious shopping mates that I too was driving an import.

The one thing about soy that troubled me was that it was often used to simulate meat. My decision to become a vegetarian was based on health reasons alone, as I harbored no ethical objection to a slab of prime rib smothered in butter. Nevertheless, I could not help feeling just a little bit hypocritical every time I choked down a soy burger. If eating meat was unhealthy or immoral, why did vegetarians seem OK with pretending to eat meat, and why was I still haunted by this vexing desire for chicken thighs? Was my weakness a sign of a wavering belief in the vegetarian faith, or was I simply experiencing a million years of evolutionary physiological conditioning?

In this brave new world of vegetarianism, where it seemed that even the soy products were substitutes for others based on soy, I drank loads of skim milk and ate plenty of fruits, vegetables and sometimes nuts. I also drank gallons of fruit juice, particularly apple juice. Before my conversion, and with the exception of orange juice, I rarely drank fruit juices, as I found them to be too sweet. But caloric balances, like matter, can neither be created nor destroyed, only changed. So in place of the fat and protein that I once consumed, I substituted prodigious amounts of carbohydrates. This was, after all, the recommended regimen of the dietary experts: increase carbohydrate intake up to sixty-five percent of daily calories, while reducing fat consumption to thirty percent or less. Most of the fat I did consume came in the form of vegetable oils.

It never occurred to me that despite my weight loss, all those carbohydrates were slowly working against me. I didn't know that many of the carbohydrates I consumed were being converted to fat. I didn't realize that the skim milk I drank was essentially a dead product, one that provided questionable nutritional benefit. I didn't understand the fact that the vegetable oils and many of the partially hydrogenated fats in the so-called lowfat products I consumed were loaded with dangerous trans fats and free radicals. I had no idea that over-consumption of soy has been linked to reduced testosterone levels in men, along with breast growth and nipple discharge.

What I did know was that even though I was thinner and looked healthier, I didn't feel healthy. Nearly a year into my low-fat vegetarian ordeal, I found that I lacked the strength to do the kind of physical activities I really enjoyed. I couldn't hike very far without becoming winded. I felt more tired than usual, so exercise was difficult. Once, on a family vacation, I accompanied my mother-in-law on a morning walk that followed a course up a steep hill. She was in her seventies at the time, almost twice my age, but I was the one who had trouble making it to the top.

What was even more troubling was the emotional cloud that darkened my perspective on everything. It seemed to shadow me wherever I went. It manifested itself as a change in mood that lay somewhere between mild discontent and outright depression. The worst of it was my new obsession with food. Every single day, I spent a good portion of my waking hours thinking about food. When would I eat my next meal? How could I doctor up a batch of tofu to make it taste like something edible? If I ate a really big salad, could I fill the hole in my stomach that daily gnawed at me, like an ulcer? What good did it do to fill up on fruits, vegetables and grain products when I was never satisfied and always hungry? I was eating right and living right, so why did it all feel so wrong?

Like my previous failed attempts at losing weight, this diet also came to an end. My fall from grace coincided with the death of my father-in-law and an unexpected encounter with a plate of chicken. I was away in California visiting family when the news came. I hurried home to Phoenix to be with my wife. Mary had gone to comfort her mother who lived some distance away, so I arrived at an empty house, exhausted from the trip made all the more difficult by a violent storm that shook up the plane as it descended into Phoenix. By the time I turned the key to the door of our house, I was anxious, saddened by the recent events. . . and extremely hungry.

Mary had been entertaining a number of nieces and nephews, all about the same age as my own children. There was ample evidence of children's play throughout the house. Not wanting to force our vegetarian beliefs on these children—all of them committed omnivores—Mary had purchased food that was more to their liking, including some fried chicken. I knew from the moment I opened the refrigerator that I was no match for the seductive platter.

I cannot recall how many pieces I ate, only that I abandoned myself to my darkest inner desires. Like the backsliding, meat-eating sinner that I was, I wallowed in my crime with a childish glee. All other concerns were forgotten. Each tasty piece of chicken was followed by a solemn vow not to touch another, which was followed by yet another succulent piece, and another vow.

Finally satiated, I sat back and patted my much reduced, post-vegetarian stomach, and smiled the smile of the contented. At the funeral, I felt guilty for feeling so good, but the sense of vitality that surged through my body was intoxicating. It took a tremendous amount of self-control to keep from grinning throughout the whole affair. Later, the rising tide of new-found energy was so overwhelming, I had to fight to keep from turning cartwheels at the cemetery. It was the first time in over a year I had felt this good. I was alive again, and I liked it.

At first, adding meat to my still mostly vegetarian diet gave me a new lease on life, but having fallen off the vegetarian wagon, I decided to roll beneath the wheels for good measure. Along with the meat, I increased my consumption of unhealthy processed foods full of trans fats, refined flour and sugar. In no time at all, I gained back all fifty pounds I had lost and quite a bit more.

LOW-CARB MANIA

I had heard about the low-carbohydrate Atkins diet but initially wrote it off as just another fad. How, I reasoned, could a man eschew fruits and vegetables, the staples of dieting, and instead gorge himself on meat of every kind and still, somehow, lose weight? This regimen made the cabbage diet seem reasonable and prudent. Yet every day I heard about some new bit of positive evidence that confirmed the validity of low-carb dieting. As media attention to the diet continued to build, my curiosity got the best of me. The clincher was the virulent reaction from the entrenched lowfat camp, which all but accused the low-carb converts of trying to commit food-induced suicide. The tenor of the attacks made me suspect that the diet might actually be effective.

Mary and I bought Dr. Atkins' book and read a few chapters—OK we read maybe one chapter and skimmed half of another. We were so excited about trying the diet that we really didn't have time to actually read the book. Eventually, we would pay for our haste. We did what I believe many people have done, we simply acted on the information gleaned from stories in the media, the gist of which was that you could eat all the meat you wanted and lose weight, so long as you never again consumed any carbohydrates. This advice, by the way, cannot be found in any book recommending a low-carb diet (Atkins recommends lots of vegetables and some fruit, especially after the first few weeks) but back in the heady days of the low-carb craze, this inaccurate description of the Atkins diet was all over the local and national news, both in the print and electronic media. So much for accurate science reporting.

The first thing we did was purchase an alarming amount of meat—beef, fowl, pork, sea food, lamb, it didn't really matter, the only prerequisite being that the day's meal must, at one time, have walked, swam or flown. I imagined barnyards across America rapidly depleted of all life.

Our meals took on the look and feel of a Paleolithic buffet, where an arugula salad was as rare as table manners at a hunter-gatherer tea party. Had we possessed the knowledge and the means to roast an entire pig and dress him up on a platter with the requisite apple in his mouth, I'm sure we would have done so. I began to feel like a character from *Clan of the Cave Bear*, my contribution to the dinner conversation devolving into rudimentary grunts of "Meat. More meat."

The amazing thing was that we actually lost weight. It felt as though we had stepped through a portal into the Bizzaro World of fad dieting, and were living every vegetarian's worst nightmare. Shopping excursions were a breeze. No longer would we tarry for hours in the produce section, squeezing tomatoes and thumping melons. We rejoiced at being set free from decisions about which nutrition-free sugared cereal to buy. Never again would we be disappointed by the pasty, flavorless taste of store-bought bread. The metallic stench of frozen foods in microwavable bags was now a thing of the past. Our rejection of carbohydrates had nearly freed us from the tyranny of shopping. In the grocery store, we had wings.

But like all bad marriages, our love affair with low-carb dieting went south soon after the honeymoon. Although I never thought it possible, I actually grew tired of eating meat. On our trips to the grocery store, I would often gaze wistfully, like a rejected lover, at the produce section on my way to the meat locker. In my dreams, ripe red tomatoes, succulent fruit and dark green leafy vegetables beckoned seductively.

To quote T.S. Eliot, the end of our low-carb diet came, "not with a bang, but a whimper." Slowly, we reverted to our old eating habits. Before we realized it, teeth-rotting, fructose-laden sodas and trans fat-laced foods were once again a part of our lives. It goes without saying that I regained the weight I had lost.

I tried dieting, tried exercising for hours each day, tried Weight Watchers, tried diet drugs, embraced vegetarianism and even wallowed in meatism, but nothing worked. I read books, following the advice of the diet gurus and purchased magazines featuring bronze, hard-bodied models on the cover and wild claims of "fast, easy" weight loss. After wading through reams of advertising for suspect dietary supplements, I found the claims to be either too difficult to duplicate, suspiciously optimistic or downright dangerous. Along the way, I kept up with the latest weight loss studies and breathless accounts of the most recent breakthrough in "blockbuster" diet pills. And yet, all I had to show for my efforts was a closet full of super-sized clothing.

What I and most Americans didn't recognize was the fact that tremendous social, political and economic changes had taken place during the previous decades. These changes would have a profound effect on the health of Americans far into the future. These changes, in fact, are still taking place. The results can be seen in the staggering statistics that track the increase in obesity, diabetes, cancer and heart disease in this country. And not just in hospitals either. On the playgrounds of America, tubby children on diabetes medication clutch sugary soda pop purchased from the school vending machines while their waistbands continue to expand.

Much has been written about how to motivate people to make positive change in their lives. I realize now that my failure at weight loss was due not to a lack of motivation, but to ignorance of the social, political and economic changes that governed American nutrition policy and determined much of what I ate.

Often, I hear from people desperate for change who say, "Just tell me what to do. Tell me what to eat." I do not doubt their sincerity, but I remind them that they are not automatons, mindless machines designed to execute orders without understanding. Real weight loss solutions can only come from a real understanding of the problem, and the problem does not begin and end with the individual. Like weeds in a garden, the problem has roots spread far beyond any individual, spread into the very foundations of our society. Government, industry and individuals all had a hand in creating this problem, and they all can have a hand in solving it. A study of the larger reasons behind why we eat and what we eat provided the knowledge I needed to unburden myself of more than one hundred fifty pounds.

To begin this study, we'll take a brief look at some of the players who have complicated our efforts to obtain better health. While they are part of the problem, they can also be part of the solution. They are the Diet Priesthood.

Part Two
Losing Our Way

Chapter Five

The Diet Priesthood
Key Players in the Cult of Dieting

Pray for deliverance.

Over the years, I have visited many doctors, due primarily to changing health plans and a move to the East Coast. Usually, during the examination, the doctors avoided the issue of my weight, as though my expanding girth were somehow invisible. More likely, they just took it for granted that this was the natural order of things for someone like me, and that they were merely playing their role, writing the requisite prescriptions and offering the cheerless pronouncement that I was "in good health." I always completed that sentence in my mind: ". . . .for someone your size." It occurred to me even then that my doctors were more focused on the symptoms of my problem than the root cause: obesity.

Whenever I ventured from the script and inquired about help for weight loss, the invariable response was either to eat less and exercise more—or try some newfangled diet drug that made big promises in the popular press but offered little beyond scary side effects once I read the fine print. Sometimes they handed me outdated brochures, which given how old they were, might as well have been printed on ancient Egyptian papyrus. Respectful as I was of professionals in white coats, and feeling completely responsible for my poor health, I never bothered to tell any of them that their advice and brochures were useless. After all, I knew I needed to eat less and exercise more and I believed that I needed to follow a lowfat diet. But what I really needed, the thing that would have been of greatest help to me, was for these learned men and women of science to explain exactly how I was to accomplish these things.

The conclusion I came to over my decade-long struggle with obesity was that all of the reputable experts were pretty much in agreement on the following basic tenets of weight loss:

- Consume fewer calories than you expend, and you will magically lose weight.
- Follow a high-carbohydrate, low-fat diet, and you will magically lose weight.
- Eat whatever you want, in moderation, and you will magically lose weight.
- Stop choosing to be fat, and you will magically lose weight.

Having followed propositions one and two for years with nothing but additional poundage to show for my efforts, I had little faith in their effectiveness. Tenet number three was patently ridiculous. How could eating candy bars for breakfast possibly help? If the obese could "eat in moderation," they wouldn't be obese, now would they? As for tenet four, I've never met anyone who wants to be fat. I took this one to be complete nonsense concocted by out-of-touch scientists and policy makers blinded by their own prejudice, a prejudice that equates obesity with sin.

There was something uncomfortably familiar about all this. One day, when I suggested that food might be the cause of a health problem that my daughter was experiencing, her doctor dismissed the notion—and me—with an impatient scowl and a wave of the hand. He would not even entertain the idea. I thought that as a man of science, he might at least consider the possibility, but he seemed positively offended by the notion. It occurred to me that the only other time I had observed this kind of blind faith in one's position was in church. Religious belief, after all, is founded on unquestioning faith, no matter how illogical the belief.

I began to see in the dietary tenets this same unwavering faith. The truth became quite clear to me. Low-fat dieting was more than just an approach to eating and nutrition, it was a cult based on unsound science. I realized that there were two types of people who remained true to this faith: the believers who practiced it, even after years of repeated failure, and those who preached the doctrine—the doctors, dieticians, and weight-loss gurus. . . the Diet Priesthood.

The diet priesthood constitutes that order of health professionals which seeks to preserve the dietary status quo. It matters not that the dietary wisdom of the last several decades has not halted the thickening of America's waistline. Their faith-based beliefs shield them from the unpleasant truth that millions of Americans must live with every day. When a member of this priesthood is confronted with a notion contrary to what he believes, he responds with ridicule. If you show him evidence that animal fat is beneficial to the human body or that consumption of processed food leads to excess insulin resulting in weight gain, he will denounce the idea while sputtering about the need for "long-term" studies and harping on the dangers of "increased risks."

THE MEDICAL PROFESSION

The medical profession harbors a large number of diet priests. These doctors have abandoned responsibility for patient care to the pharmaceutical industry. Almost none has received adequate nutrition training in medical school. In fact, many understand less about the connection between diet and health than their obese patients. They turn a blind eye to the core cause of obesity—our modern diet—and instead hype expensive drugs and treatments that only manage and maintain the symptoms. The result is a steady stream of medical insurance reimbursements for them and years of suffering for their patients.

Doctors used to look at each patient as an individual, each with a unique set of problems to diagnose and treat with the appropriate medical solution. No longer. Many doctors today practice a type of treatment model similar to a paint-by-numbers hobby kit, where patient treatment conforms to a well-established template, whether it works or not. The irony is that some doctors struggle with the very same weight problems as their patients, yet feel compelled to promote a treatment model at which they themselves have failed.

THE PHARMACEUTICAL INDUSTRY

In *The Truth About the Drug Companies: How They Deceive Us and What To Do About It*, author Marcia Angell, MD, reveals the ugly underside of one of the world's most profitable industries. The pharmaceutical industry privatizes taxpayer-funded government research and then makes billions pedaling their drugs to American consumers at some of the highest prices in the world. Like a virus invading the body of modern medicine, pharmaceutical reps fan out across the country, acting as ghost doctors through their influence on your health care provider. Many doctors naively believe that their prescribing patterns are unaffected by the soft money that flows from Big Pharma to Big Medicine. But these days, sound science and the search for truth compete with the never-ending quest for increased revenues and bigger profits. This trend toward checkbook science contributes to a culture of biased medical research that exaggerates the positive outcomes of industry-funded studies, while down playing or ignoring negative side effects.

After college, in the early 1980s, I worked as a medical and graphic illustrator for a large hospital in the southwest. One of my duties was to assist doctors with developing displays to present the results of their research. These displays typically included poster-sized photographs, illustrations, text and charts. Sometimes the research results for a particular body of work were insignificant. This fact was revealed when blown up to poster size and presented as a chart. It was not uncommon for the doctor to request a reworked chart that exaggerated the increments of the x or y axis in order to exaggerate the research results. This was always explained away as "making the results easier to see." While technically true, we all knew that it was also a way to spin the results to make them appear more meaningful than they actually were.

As factions within the medical industry continue to redefine formerly healthy populations as sick and in need of medication, more and more people are caught up in the net—including children. The goal is to expand the market for medication to healthy populations previously beyond consideration for drug treatment. Two examples of this trend are blood pressure and cholesterol levels. In both cases, the risk point has been revised steadily downward, converting previously healthy people into patients needing prescription drugs. Crime may not pay, but medicating healthy populations certainly does.

What of the Food and Drug Administration? It is the consensus of many drug industry watchdogs that the FDA sees the drug industry as a client rather than as an industry that needs to be watched.

THE FOOD INDUSTRY

To satiate our need for the new and different and the industry's need for more sources of profit, the food companies dump thousands of new products on our supermarket shelves each year. Once you get beyond the basics of meat, seafood, fruits, vegetables and dairy products, you enter the realm of processed foods. These foods are designed to appeal to our senses with their tastes, smells and textures, but beneath their superficial exteriors, they are little more than calorie-dense, nutrient-poor "lab experiments" designed to keep us coming back for more.

Under the guise of convenience, the ever expanding prepared foods sector of the food industry has sold us a bill of goods. With convenience and pricing driving consumer purchases on the buy side, and cold, hard profits driving corporate practices on the sell side, personal health runs a distant third in the race to determine what will be available at the grocery store. In short, modern foods have become the real weapons of mass destruction. The American Dietetic Association carries the flag for the processed food industry by promoting the consumption of junk foods as "part of a healthy diet." This is not surprising: the ADA receives funding from several sectors of the processed food industry.

Laws governing the health claims that food manufacturers can make have been relaxed under the Bush administration. As with the drug industry, the FDA rarely intervenes on behalf of the citizens it is supposed to protect. In this industry-friendly environment, one popular fried chicken retailer even aired television commercials touting its product as "healthy." Even leaders within the advertising industry—an industry not usually shy about making outrageous claims—were appalled. The ads were mercifully withdrawn after a short run.

THE RADICAL FUNDAMENTALISTS

A relatively new branch of the priesthood has emerged in recent years, thanks to the Internet. An offshoot, or splinter cell, of the food industry, they fulfill the role of attack dog and are more militant in their approach. Like all fundamentalist organizations that employ fear as their primary weapon, these groups engage in wholesale scare mongering to advance their agenda. Funded and supported by legitimate food manufacturers, wholesalers and retailers, these groups operate under jingoistic monikers, with names like "Consumer Coalition for Free Choice" and "Citizen's Group for Freedom." Their target: the infidels, that is anyone who disparages any food as unhealthy. Infidels must be publicly ridiculed lest the general public listen to what they say.

In their writings the fundamentalists tend to rely heavily on terms of abuse like "food cop" and "food nanny," and for some reason they are inexplicably fond of the word "tasty."

THE WEIGHT LOSS INDUSTRY

This group is populated by diet book writers, exercise equipment salesmen and diet supplement manufacturers. Their qualifications in the fields of nutrition, diet and human physiology run the gamut from knowledgeable to laughable. As an example of the latter, not long ago a certain well-known diet guru claimed on national television that the human brain needs five hundred grams of carbohydrates per day. A tame "medical expert" in attendance eagerly nodded in agreement. Millions of viewers were left ignorant of the fact that the human brain can function quite well with little or no carbohydrates in the diet at all.

Chapter Five: The Diet Priesthood

. . . .

Of all the groups that make up the priesthood, this order is the most quick-acting. Once they get a sense that money can be made on a new fad, their manufacturing machines are retooled and up and running in no time. Announce on Monday a new study showing that a chemical substance derived from decades-old fruitcake results in weight loss, and the books, CDs and supplements extolling fruit cake derivatives will be available for sale by Friday.

YOU AND ME

Of course, I can't lay all the blame for our predicament at the feet of government and industry. Sure, we've been fooled, bamboozled, led astray and even lied to by industry and government special interests, but in the end, each of us is responsible for his own life. As long as we cling to a blind faith that leads us to accept whatever we are told, we are complicit. When we fail to learn about our own bodies, to cook our own food or to think for ourselves, we are complicit. When industry says we can eat gobs of sugary, lowfat foods without any ill effect, and we accept that claim without question, we are complicit. When we allow family farmers to be driven off the land and replaced by factory farms, we are complicit. When corporations and the health care industry bring us the next miracle weight loss drug, and we accept it without question, we are complicit. When we stand idly by as science is co-opted by corporate dollars and blindly accept the resulting "checkbook" science as sound, we are complicit. And when we allow the food, fashion, entertainment and advertising industries to tell our children what to think, do and be, we are complicit in the demise of our children and ourselves.

THE HERETICS

Fortunately, there are heretics within all of the above groups. These are the unbelievers who go their own way, practicing a Socratic philosophy that challenges conventional wisdom and adheres to the Hippocratic dictate: First do no harm. They are doctors, medical researchers, nutritionists, authors, food producers and consumers—perhaps even your next door neighbor. Seek them out and support them in their efforts.

A short list of brave heretics includes nutrition researcher, Sally Fallon, author of *Nourishing Traditions*, arguably the best cookbook ever written; Mary Enig, PhD, who tells the truth about fat in her book, *Know Your Fats: The Complete Primer for Understanding the Nutrition of Fats, Oils and Cholesterol*; Uffe Ravnskov, MD PhD, author of *The Cholesterol Myths*; Marion Nestle, author of *Food Politics*, which exposes the Machiavellian politics that gave us our current food policy; and, most important, the late Dr. Weston A. Price, DDS, author of *Nutrition and Physical Degeneration*, an account of his ground-breaking research on the principles of healthy diets among non-industrialized people.

Change is difficult. For some industries and professions, it is downright unprofitable. Thus, resistance to the idea that conventional dietary wisdom is flawed will undoubtedly continue. Having lost faith in modern dietary wisdom, I have found a new belief system that actually works. That belief system is one based on traditional foods: grass-fed natural meats including organ meats, plenty of animal fats, old-fashioned cod liver oil, wild seafood, organic fruits, vegetables and nuts, whole grains and healthful raw dairy products. These are the heretical foods that brought me back from the brink of self-destruction.

Why do we do it? Why do we take on the burden of foods that are clearly unhealthy? Why did we stop cooking our own food? When it comes to our consumer behavior, why do we do the things we do?

Chapter Six

Consumer Engineering and Why We Buy

How we have been trained to buy products and services, whether we need them or not

When it comes to making sense of your shopping behavior, telephones and food have more in common than you may realize. I'll explain in a moment, but first I want to review one of my favorite children's stories, Pinocchio. Yes, your phone company, the food industry and Pinocchio are all relevant to the question of why you can no longer fit into last year's pants.

In the modernized version of Pinocchio, we have the story of a wooden puppet who wants to be a real boy. The question is, why does Pinocchio want to be real anyway? As a puppet, he can walk and talk and go to school and even learn to read. In fact, in practically every way he can already do what any real boy can do, so what is it that drives Pinocchio? I believe it is the same thing that drives all of us.

It has been said that the story of Pinocchio is really a story about the transition from adolescence to adulthood. In most versions, Pinocchio is continually manipulated by the characters he meets and these encounters always end in disaster. Very often, Pinocchio is the chief architect of his own misfortunes, but regardless of how he gets into trouble, the one common theme is that Pinocchio lacks the maturity and the ability to direct and control his future. That shouldn't surprise us, because he is, after all, a puppet, and puppets have no self control. And while there are no physical strings that direct his behavior, metaphorically Pinocchio is still bound by his inability to think for himself. It isn't until Pinocchio learns to think and make decisions based on something beyond his own selfish and misguided desires that he is released from his prison of strings. We come to see in a very concrete way the notion that Pinocchio represents all of us in our very human struggle for self-determination.

The level of self-determination we have—that is, the perceived and genuine ability to chart our own course—is one of the ways in which we judge the quality of our freedom. Few components of social life are more abhorrent than the sense that we are not in control of our own destiny. When we lose this sense of control over our future, we often rebel, but just as often we become paralyzed by hopelessness. Yet the need to be in control of our own lives is so strong that even the illusion of control is preferable to the stark realization that we, like Pinocchio, are mere puppets of a larger, unseen hand that determines our fate.

CONSUMERS MADE TO ORDER

Whenever I talk about the role of consumer engineering in the evolution of how and what we eat, two of the most common responses are shock and disbelief. Many people are shocked at the idea that much of what we know, or think we know, about food and nutrition may not be based solely on the issue of health.

The more common response is disbelief. Some very intelligent people simply cannot comprehend a world in which their thoughts and beliefs about food are not their own. They bristle at the mere suggestion that they may have been manipulated in some way, that their beliefs about food have been engineered as part of some grand, decades-long campaign to make them "better consumers of convenience foods."

In the past, I found it difficult to make a convincing case for the idea that some of our beliefs and behaviors concerning food are, in fact, not of our own making. It is a task akin to convincing someone who has never seen an elephant that such creatures really do exist. Without an actual elephant, or at least a picture of one, to submit as proof of their existence, incredulity prevails.

Chapter Six: Consumer Engineering and Why We Buy

. . . .

Proving the existence of elephants and other oddities of the physical world is quite simple today thanks to the modern miracle of digital photography. But how do you demonstrate to someone that some of their most cherished beliefs such as, "I don't have time to cook," are more a fabrication of clever marketing than a reflection of reality? My mother had five children and my wife's mother had twelve. Both of these women worked outside the home and were extremely busy, even by today's standards. How was it possible, then, in an age before the proliferation of microwave ovens, pizza delivery and the avalanche of convenience foods that we have today, that they were able to cook real food and put dinner on the table for their families? Even in the face of numberless examples such as these, many people still cling to the belief that for the first time in human history, we are too busy to prepare our own food.

The problem, of course, is that we are all victims of consumer engineering. Some of our beliefs about food and nutrition are actually the product of food industry strategy campaigns, often carried out decades ago. Because these changes in opinion took place over a number of decades, it is difficult for many people to perceive them.

I had been searching for a way to describe the phenomenon of consumer engineering when a cab driver revealed the solution. He was a talkative fellow who spent the nearly one-hour ride discussing the foibles of his family. As an example, he told me his wife had given him a mobile phone for his birthday. She had taken advantage of one of those two-for-one phone giveaways that you can't seem to escape from nowadays. The problem was, he already had a mobile phone. What his wife had given him was a new monthly bill, not a gift.

I understood immediately what his wife had not comprehended. Though she had saved a few dollars on a phone her husband didn't even need her family would be saddled with monthly bill payments. These payments represented an added and unnecessary expense to their household budget. She might just as well have made a voluntary monthly donation to the phone company. From the description that her husband gave, she sounded like a delightful woman, bright and resourceful.

How then could she have made such a bad business deal? How did she rationalize her husband's need for a phone when he already had one? Where did she think the extra money to pay for a new phone was going to come from?

On the train, on the bus, on the street, at weddings and funerals, in church and even in public rest rooms, mobile phones are everywhere. From eight-year-olds to octogenarians, everyone has a phone these days. If cell phones had existed in the late 1800s, French sculptor Auguste Rodin might well have named "The Thinker" "The Talker," perhaps posing him with a phone cupped to his ear and his mouth wide open.

I've had people tell me they can't live without their phones and more and more people are replacing their traditional land lines with mobiles. Parents all across the country are opening their monthly statements and wailing over their children's three-figure phone charges, then weeping at the loss of their retirement and children's college contributions as they dutifully pay the bill. And it isn't just a matter of technological change: the telecommunications industry is quite literally changing the behavior inherent in communication. Oddly, while mobile phones were supposed to bring us closer together, they are quite literally pulling us apart. I've seen couples on dates where one or both of them are talking on a phone and completely ignoring each other!

How is it that mankind has existed on this planet for millions of years without the need to be in constant communication, while today many people seem practically addicted to their mobile phones? The answer is consumer engineering. Just ten short years ago, almost no one had a mobile phone. How did the telecom industry engineer such a dramatic change in the way we communicate in such a short period of time? They did it through intense and clever marketing. Once you accept the fact that the telecom industry has changed the way we talk to each other in little more than a decade, it seems quite reasonable to acknowledge that the food industry could do the same thing over the course of several decades.

So what are some of the parallels between the two industries? First, cost. Mobile phones are marketed as better and more economical, and while it is true that the price of mobile phones has steadily declined, these declining costs only create an illusion of savings. In fact, mobile phones tend to be more expensive due to the complicated pricing structure of the plans, aggressive marketing schemes that package multiple phones and target teenagers, over-consumption of phone services and the often mysterious charges that are included in the typical phone bill.

Much of the same can be said for ready-to-eat convenience foods. While they are generally less expensive than higher quality whole foods, this too is an illusion when you consider the fact that we end up eating more of them. And because these foods are nutritionally poor, any gains in near-term economic savings are offset by long-term losses in health, a lower quality of life and the inevitable medical costs.

Here's another similarity: cell phone companies offer an unlimited array of phone models, features and calling plans. Despite this apparent range of choices, the quality of the phones and their performance often fails to meet expectations. Dropped calls, grainy connections and unexplained failures are just some of the unadvertised features of today's mobile phones. Oddly, while they may be quite good at taking pictures and playing MP3s, many of today's mobiles fail to match the connection quality of a rotary-dial land line phone from decades earlier.

Convenience foods are similar. While there is much to choose from, the quality leaves plenty to be desired when compared to fresh, whole foods. Much of the decline in quality comes from declining manufacturing standards and an industry obsession with profits. In an era of shrinking margins, how does the food industry convince us to pay for more lower quality food? In a word, marketing.

Ad campaigns for phones often include terms like "free," "most reliable," "flexible" and "unlimited." These powerful words are paired with images of smiling, ethnically diverse groups of attractive people, all enjoying life, ostensibly because of their phones. Now compare those ads with ads for food. Again we find images of happy people bonding at a fast food restaurant while words like "value," "family," "sale" and "quality" complete the implied message: eating certain foods or patronizing certain restaurants will improve your life. We see images of responsible, middle-class moms who gaze contentedly while their cherub-faced children happily gorge themselves on candied cereals, imitation cheese and french fries. We want to be happy like the people in the advertisements, so we willingly buy the products.

Food manufacturers know that we often base our decisions to buy certain foods on taste, cost and convenience rather than on nutritional quality, and that's what they give us. One of the principal factors that plays into phone and food purchases is "image"—how we see ourselves and how we hope others will see us if we buy a particular product. This is standard practice in the world of advertising and should surprise no one, but what is surprising is the degree to which repeated exposure to these messages tends to modify our behavior and shape our opinions. Our opinions should result from our own thoughtful analysis, not from a carefully crafted, industry-driven promotional campaign.

For most of our marriage, Mary and I chose to spend a large portion of our food budget at restaurants and in the purchase of convenience foods. Despite the fact that we were well-educated, had only two children, were blessed with flexible working hours, enjoyed all of the modern technological conveniences and grew up in households that cherished the art of cooking, we somehow managed to buy into the proposition that cooking was a tedious and time-consuming affair, one that was beneath our dignity and simply did not fit into our busy schedules.

Fortunately for us, ignorance is only a temporary condition, easily remedied by a willingness to open one's mind and think. We discovered that the reason we didn't cook was because we saw little value in it. Every day we were directly or indirectly exposed to the message that food purchases should be based on taste, cost and convenience, that we were simply too busy to make intelligent decisions about what we ate, and that we should leave those decisions to the faceless corporations that made things like yogurt in a tube and TV dinners for the microwave. Once we dared to challenge these entrenched beliefs, we realized that the primary factor governing our food purchases should be nutritional quality. Since our parents had managed to provide delicious meals year after year on a fraction of the income that we had, we concluded that we could do the same.

We took a hard look at our beliefs about food and nutrition and found that those beliefs benefited food manufactures more than they did ourselves. We saw that most of the food available at the grocery store was grain-based, filled with sugar, laced with additives, and highly processed. It made business sense for food companies to tout them as better for us and price them so as to make them irresistible.

Why does the food industry resist even a modest effort to provide healthier food? Because such a revolutionary step would raise consumer awareness. If even ten percent of consumers switched from prepared foods to whole foods, the effect on the food industry would be devastating. In fact, in order to remain viable, the prepared foods industry has to demonize cooking, telling us over and over again that we are simply too busy to cook.

Mary and I soon discovered that we had plenty of time to shop for better quality food and plenty of time to prepare it. It was all a matter of readjusting our priorities. We had surrendered to others the most critical decisions affecting our health. By paying closer attention to what we eat, and by making time for food in our lives, we have freed ourselves from the burden of poor health. Just like triumphant Pinocchio, we have refused to be misguided by others, and instead have learned to recognize the value of real self-determination.

Chapter Seven

The Trojan Horse Diet
What if some of the "healthy" foods you're eating
are doing you the most harm?

We owe a great debt of gratitude to Dr. Weston A. Price for his contribution to the study of human nutrition. Dr. Price was a dentist who in the 1930s and 1940s traveled to remote areas of the globe and discovered key principles about traditional diets. As a dentist, Dr. Price was principally concerned with the connection between diet and dental health. What he uncovered was the connection between the increasing industrialization of the food supply and the physical degeneration of the populations who consumed this food, manifested in rampant tooth decay, narrowed jaws and crooked teeth (which he called "dental deformation") in the next generation.

Accompanied by his wife and the occasional guide, Dr. Price traveled from isolated villages nestled in the Swiss Alps, to hardy communities of Eskimos in the wilderness of Alaska. In Polynesia, Africa, Australia and many other out-of-the way communities, he discovered the same connection between food and health. In a general sense, his discovery can be summed up quite simply. When isolated people adhere to their traditional diets, their health and quality of life are far better than after adopting a modern diet high in refined grains, sugar and other processed foods. The problem gets worse with succeeding generations that grow up on a modern diet. They experience advanced tooth decay, physical deformities (which first manifest as narrow dental pallets and crooked teeth), a loss of overall vigor, decreased resistance to disease and a lower quality of life. Dr. Price documented his research in his life-changing book, *Nutrition and Physical Degeneration*, a stunning account—in words and pictures—of what happens when diet goes awry.

A key finding of his research was that foods like liver, organ meats, fish eggs, fish liver oil, and eggs and butter from pastured animals, foods containing high levels of vitamins A and D, and were consumed in large amounts by healthy non-industrialized peoples; in fact, they valued these foods as sacred, especially for pregnant women and growing children. These life-giving foods are the very foods now condemned by the diet priesthood.

The physical degeneration that Dr. Price observed in the first half of the last century began with the advent of processed food and continues to the present. In fact, the chronic diseases associated with civilization—heart disease, diabetes, obesity and cancer—plague us even more greatly today, despite our advanced knowledge of human physiology and the slew of drugs and treatments we use to control them. This rise in chronic disease exactly parallels the increasing industrialization of our food supply.

Of course, environmental pollutants and destructive choices of lifestyle also contribute to our declining health, but the foods we eat, the foods that literally become a part of us, are the primary contributors to the breakdown of the human body. Our modern diet of processed, easy-open, labor-saving, pre-cooked, just-add-water, fat-free convenience foods seem like a huge step forward. We have been freed from the "tyranny" of cooking, but at what price?

FACTORY FARMS

In 1906, American writer Upton Sinclair published *The Jungle*, a scathing exposé of the American meat-packing industry. Sinclair's vivid portrayal of unsanitary and morally bankrupt slaughterhouse practices brought about sweeping changes within the meat industry. We can all breathe easier now knowing that the corrupt practices of early twentieth century America are behind us—or can we?

Chapter Seven: The Trojan Horse Diet

. . . .

Our meat is more regulated and presumably cleaner today than it was in Sinclair's era, but what do we really know about where our food comes from? Advertisements for dairy products show contented cows lolling in verdant fields beneath tranquil skies. Promotions for meat products often avoid showing the actual animals, lest we accidentally make the connection between that cute calf or pig and the pork chop or slice of veal on our dinner plate. For several generations now, we have been literally and figuratively cut off from our food, but as we have seen, it wasn't always that way.

The truth is, today's factory farms engage in practices similar to those Upton Sinclair wrote about. Dairy cows are held in confinement conditions and forced to stand on concrete floors their whole lives. They live in cathedral-sized metal sheds that enshrine man's inhumanity to animals. To keep the milk flowing, these animals receive an unnatural diet of grain, soy, bakery waste and swill from ethanol production. The cows have been selectively bred to have enormous udders; they deliver far more milk than Mother Nature ever intended. On some farms, growth hormones like BST (bovine somatotropin) are used to stimulate higher levels of milk production. Not surprisingly, these animals often get sick and are kept "productive" courtesy of a strenuous course of antibiotics. One particularly nasty illness called mastitis, an infection of the udder, is pandemic in confinement dairies. The infected animal may secrete pus into her milk, resulting in a sub-standard product that must be filtered and pasteurized before your child can drink it with any assurance of safety.

Pigs and chickens have not been excluded from the misery. Pigs are held in conditions so stressful and crowded that they engage in the practice of chewing each other's tails. Industry's response to this problem is not to reduce the number of pigs on a farm, or increase the acreage to accommodate them, but to chop off their tails! Meanwhile, biochemists are trying to breed the stress gene out of the pigs so that they'll suffer their fate without resistance.

Industrial agriculture has turned chickens into egg and meat machines, confined in cages with barely enough room for them to move around. The taste of chicken today can't compare to the taste I recall as a child. In those days, the meat was firm and flavorful and the bones quite hard. Today, meat from grocery store chickens is distastefully mealy, and the bones are soft. The commercial eggs have pale anemic yolks, inferior in taste to the delicious, deep yellow yolks from pastured chickens on a more natural diet.

Besides the illness and stress these animals suffer, the humans who live with and near them must deal with another problem: what to do with all the waste? As you might imagine, the accumulated waste produced by too many animals in too small a space produces smells so bad it makes people sick. The waste is held in onsite containment ponds. A recent news article describes how the wall of a containment pond gave way, causing a massive spill. Thousands of gallons of putrid sludge poured into a drainage ditch and eventually made its way into a nearby river, killing thousands of fish.

Factory farming taints everything it touches: animals, farm workers, environment, food, and those who consume it.

THE MODERN TRADITIONAL DIET

The healthy indigenous people that Dr. Price studied consumed a traditional diet devoid of refined and processed food. What constitutes a traditional diet? Today, many children begin their lives on soymilk before graduating to soda, sometimes while they're still on the bottle. A traditional diet does not necessarily refer, then, to the first food you eat. To understand what is meant by a traditional diet, we must first define the word "food." Eating wisely requires us to know what is in our food and what effect it will have on our long-term health. We also need to distinguish between "food" and "real food." Generally speaking, most people define food as anything we eat for nourishment, energy or the simple desire to satisfy our hunger. This is a broad definition, as you'll see, because people are remarkably adaptable with regard to what they'll eat.

I knew a kid in grade school who was particularly fond of that white crafts paste we used in school. He would snitch great gobs of the stuff and eat it surreptitiously when the teacher wasn't looking. In some parts of the world, eating dirt is not uncommon. Some people have even been known to consume objects like nuts and bolts. Most of us would not consider paste or a three-quarter inch lug nut as food, so let's refine our definition a bit more.

Food is any edible substance from a natural plant or animal source consumed for the purpose of providing nourishment and energy. This is a better description, but let's examine it further. *Real* food is food that has been minimally processed and retains its natural life-giving properties.

Most of the added ingredients in today's food are unnecessary for human nourishment. In some cases, they may even be harmful. These additives exist for three reasons, none of which has anything to do with nourishing the human body. The first is to mimic freshness by artificially extending the shelf life of the food. Without these additives, many foods would quickly go stale and rot. The second reason is that many commercially produced foods simply don't taste very good, so additives are used to enhance flavor as well as visual appeal. The third is that manufacturers are always looking for ways to cut costs and increase profits.

Artificial food additives reduce cost by replacing real ingredients with fake ones. Generally speaking, the fewer additives and preservatives a food contains, the more real it is.

The way foods are produced also determines how real they are. Beef from a cow that has been raised in abusive conditions on a diet of grains, growth hormones and antibiotics is not the same as beef from a healthy grass-fed cow. Packaged foods that have been sterilized, synthesized, homogenized, colorized, pasteurized, emulsified, flavored, pulverized, deodorized, irradiated and genetically modified do not qualify as real food. Artificially flavored and colored "yogurt" that does not require refrigeration and comes in a squeezable tube is an extreme example of this type of not-real food. "Beef" ribs made from soy is another.

Manufacturers are the primary beneficiaries of this type of not-real food production. Consumers lose because eating substances that are foreign and possibly harmful to the human body, and produced in a manner inconsistent with good nutrition, leads to the ruin of our health.

Real food, then, can be defined as food that contains few or no additives or artificial ingredients. Real food nourishes, builds and energizes the body and is produced in a manner consistent with retaining the life-giving properties of the food. Everything from salads to pizza made from real ingredients qualifies as real food. These are the traditional foods that have nourished humanity down through the ages. It follows, then, that a traditional diet is one comprised of real foods that are in harmony with the evolutionary physiology of the human body.

A DIETARY ODYSSEY

Two of my favorite stories growing up were Homer's twin epics, the *Iliad* and the *Odyssey*. They tell the story of the long Trojan War, and of the Greek hero Odysseus' even longer journey home. I was especially fascinated by the Trojan horse, a "gift" from the Greeks that turned out to be the instrument of the Trojans' defeat. Today, poor dietary advice has turned out to be a Trojan horse in the lives of many unsuspecting people. For decades, we have been at war with our cultural and culinary history, traditional foods and, in particular, dietary fats. Fat, especially saturated fat, has been the scapegoat for all that is wrong with what America eats. The oft repeated warning to "eat lowfat," has become more than just a cornerstone of nutritional dogma—it has become sacred scripture, constantly preached by the diet priesthood to millions of faithful adherents.

We have adopted a nutritional belief system that demonizes fat with the fervor of religious zealotry. It is a faith we practice daily, making fat-free food choices with a numbing sense of duty, one that approaches fundamentalist fanaticism. We have been taught that salvation and thin thighs can only be attained by a strict adherence to a fat-free lifestyle, and so, without question, we blindly sacrifice our bodies, our minds—and our children—to this belief.

Yet despite an almost universal belief in lowfat dieting, most of us end up with weight gain, illness and premature death. Although obesity, heart disease, diabetes, allergies, asthma and fatigue befall us anyway, we soldier on, obediently invoking protection against the evil of dietary fat, while we medicate ourselves into oblivion.

WHAT ARE WE REALLY EATING?

The image of Americans as lazy gluttons stuffing themselves with prodigious amounts of dietary animal fat is a gross exaggeration. The following statistics from the *USDA Food Consumption, Prices, and Expenditures* report reveals what Americans really eat. Except where noted, the report covers the period between 1970 and 1997.

Although per capita consumption of meat of all types reached near record high levels in 1994, the proportion of fat from meat declined from thirty-five percent in 1970 to twenty-five percent in 1994. Saturated fat consumption fell from thirty-seven percent to twenty-six percent. In 1960, beef producers began raising leaner beef by moving away from the traditionally fatter and tastier breeds, like Herefords and Angus. The trends are similar for pork. While overall consumption increased slightly from 1970 to 1998, the meat was much leaner, reflecting consumer trends toward lowfat eating. In all, per capita meat consumption, including red meat, poultry and fish, was up about thirteen pounds per year, but this change was due mostly to an increase in poultry consumption. Consumption of red meat, which was significantly leaner and contained much less saturated fat, actually declined.

During this period, shell eggs, once considered a perfect food, saw a per capita decline from two hundred seventy-six to one hundred seventy-three eggs per year, due to consumer fear of cholesterol. Between 1970 and 1994, daily consumption of cholesterol declined thirteen percent, from four hundred seventy to four hundred ten milligrams per day. Yet heart disease remains at epidemic levels.

In the dairy category, whole milk consumption decreased by two-thirds between 1970 and 1997. This decrease was offset by America's love affair with cheese and fluid cream products. Average consumption of cheese increased one hundred forty-six percent! Lest you think Americans inexplicably evolved into connoisseurs of fine gourmet cheeses, think again. Most of that cheese—up to two-thirds—came packaged as convenience food in the form of pizza, snack foods, fast food sandwiches, chips, bagel spreads, etc. While cheese is a high-fat item, when it comes as convenience food it is accompanied by prodigious amounts of grains, sugars and processed vegetable oils.

Consumption of fluid cream products increased from just under ten half-pints to seventeen half-pints, usually in the form of ice cream and dips, while overall fluid butterfat consumption (in whole and reduced-fat milk and cream) declined by thirty-seven percent.

Surprisingly, in 1997 Americans on average consumed fifty-seven pounds more fruit and eighty-seven pounds more vegetables than in 1970. Given all the finger wagging from health experts, you would never guess that produce consumption has risen so much.

The most startling figures in the USDA report come in the categories of grain, sugar and "fat and oils." American consumption of flour and cereal products increased from one hundred thirty-six pounds in 1970 to a whopping two hundred pounds in 1997. That's a lot of dough. Much of this increase came in the form of fast food and snack food such as pizza, pasta, crackers, chips and—the mother of all grain foods—ready-to-eat cereals. Breakfast cereal consumption between 1980 and 1997 increased by forty-one percent to seventeen pounds per person per year! Much of that cereal was consumed with mounds of sugar. In fact, in 1997, our consumption of sugars—table sugar and high-fructose corn syrup (HFCS)—rose twenty-eight percent, or thirty-four pounds per person, to a total of one hundred fifty-four pounds of the sweet stuff. That's fifty-three teaspoons—almost two cups—per day! A far cry from the six to eighteen teaspoons (based on a diet of sixteen hundred to twenty-eight hundred calories) our government recommends in the Food Guide Pyramid. The use of corn sweeteners, especially HFCS, skyrocketed due to favorable government agricultural policies toward corn growers and an overabundant supply.

One place these corn sweeteners wound up in was beverages. In 1986, the average American swilled twenty-eight gallons of carbonated soda. By 1997, that number had increased to forty-one gallons, a forty-seven percent increase. Soda has replaced milk as the drink—or drug—of choice among children and teenagers.

Finally, let's look at fats and oils. Unless you live in some kind of lumberjack commune or South Sea island, it's unlikely that you know anyone who cooks with lard, tallow, coconut or palm oil. Even the use of butter is a rarity today. Between 1970 and 1997, consumption of animal fats declined by a fourth while consumption of polyunsaturated vegetable fats increased by two-fifths. During this same period, consumption of polyunsaturated salad and cooking oils jumped from fifteen to twenty-nine pounds per capita!

Experts like Mary Enig, PhD, have warned the public about the fact that polyunsaturated vegetable oils can become oxidized quite easily, forming free radicals that cause cancer and atherosclerosis in humans. Unfortunately, since the 1950s, health "experts" have been advising us to consume polyunsaturated oils as a preventative measure against heart disease and cancer. These rancid oils are, in fact, more likely to create health problems than prevent them. Government policy also promotes the consumption of partially hydrogenated vegetable fats, which are engineered to behave like saturated fat. These products, in the form of margarine and shortening, are loaded with harmful trans fats. Baked goods—including cookies, cakes and crackers—peanut butter, fried foods, soups and cereals are all loaded with trans fats. Commercial salad dressings contain both liquid oils and partially hydrogenated oils. We eat far more of these dressings today than we did thirty years ago because we are following the advice to eat more salads! A USDA survey showed that between 1989 and 1991, the average woman between the ages of nineteen and fifty obtained more vegetable fat from salad dressing than anything else she was eating.

Changes in U.S. Per Capita Food Consumption, 1970 - 1997

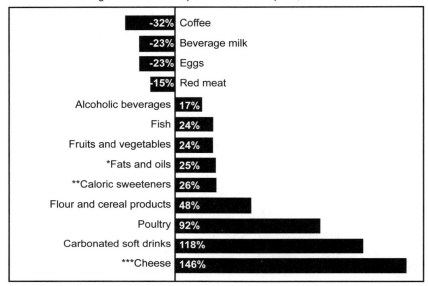

Source: *USDA Economic Research Service*
*   Represents added fats and oils (shortening, margarine, vegetable oil, butter) found in fried foods, snack foods and salad dressing. Excludes natural fats found in foods like milk and meat. By 1994, these fats and oils contributed to 52% of total fat intake. Meat, fish, and poultry followed with 25% of the total.
**   Includes caloric sweeteners used in soft drinks.
***   Two-thirds of cheese consumption came in the form of prepared foods.

Trends in Obesity from 1976 - 2000

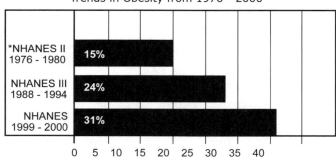

Source: Derived from the CDC and the National Center for Health Statistics
*   National Health and Nutrition Examination Survey, age-adjusted by the direct method to U.S. Census Bureau estimates for the year 2000 using the age groups 20-29, 40-59 and 60-74 years.

Chapter Seven: The Trojan Horse Diet

. . . .

OBESITY AND HEART DISEASE

It is interesting to note the changes in the health of Americans over the same time period as the food consumption survey. According to the 1999-2000 National Health and Nutrition Examination Survey conducted by a division of the Centers for Disease Control, rates of obesity doubled between 1976 and 2000. Heart disease continues as the number one killer in America, racking up almost nine hundred fifty thousand lives in the year 2000, according to the American Heart Association. While the death rate from heart disease has declined slightly due to improvements in treatment, Americans continue to be stricken by this killer in astounding numbers.

When I look at these statistics, I see a reflection of myself. Just like many other Americans, I followed the prevailing health advice. I ate more fruits and vegetables and less fat, and abandoned whole milk and eggs. I substituted poultry cooked in polyunsaturated oils for red meat and replaced butter with margarine. I consumed prodigious amounts of sweetener in soda, fruit juices and just about ninety percent of the convenience foods on my grocery store shelf. I didn't smoke, drink alcohol or consume coffee. In short, I did just about everything the experts said I should, but despite my virtuous life, I still managed to gain over two hundred pounds.

What I didn't know was that the polyunsaturated vegetable oils and partially hydrogenated fats that had replaced the animal fats in my diet were destroying my health. I didn't know that my lowfat diet was actually kindling my appetite to eat more. I never realized that a diet high in grains, sugars and supposedly healthier vegetable oil was actually a Trojan horse, piling on the pounds faster than I could exercise them off. I didn't know that the reason I failed at dieting so often was because the food I ate was grossly insufficient to meet my nutritional needs. I didn't know that bingeing and devouring an entire family-sized bag of potato chips was a sign that my body was craving healthy fat. I didn't know that those late-night eating marathons could have been completely avoided had I simply added a little healthy fat in the form of a steak, some coconut oil or butter to my diet. In the end, I didn't know that my inability to exercise regularly had more to do with a series of diets insufficient to sustain me physically and mentally. There was a lot I didn't know, and apparently none of my doctors knew anything either.

Dietary animal fat has been pegged as the primary culprit in the long-running siege against our health. However, when you review the USDA statistics, you can see that while consumption of saturated fat has decreased overall, consumption of processed convenience foods has increased dramatically. Is it really that difficult to see the connection between these so-called foods and the increase in heart disease, obesity and diabetes?

It is a well-established fact that obesity is a risk factor for heart disease. When many consumers began to reduce their intake of sweeteners and grains, our government sponsored a number of studies intended to refute low-carb dieting. Instead, these studies proved the connection between excess refined carbohydrates and obesity. Is it not reasonable to suggest that heart disease, which correlates with obesity, may be connected to the excess starches and sugars found in processed foods? Why then is the scientific community still obsessed with saturated fats?

I don't mean to suggest that the Western diet is the sole cause of heart disease. Smoking, stress and physical inactivity play key roles as well. What I do say is that much evidence exists to challenge the theory that cholesterol and saturated fat cause heart disease. So much evidence, in fact, that one begins to wonder where, exactly, the science behind the theory can be found? It almost seems as though the proponents of the diet-heart hypothesis are operating more on their personal faith in the theory than on scientific fact. Despite their protestations in favor of "sound science," they are more like faith healers than scientists.

As the truth about dietary fat emerges, and we begin to reapply the wisdom of our ancestors, we can celebrate a long-awaited homecoming. Like Odysseus, the road home to wellness may be long and difficult, but Odysseus finally made it. I found that once I mustered the courage to plot my own course home, I could make it, too.

Chapter Seven: The Trojan Horse Diet

· ·

THE DIETARY DARK AGES

For the last few decades, I've lived through a personal and public dark age of nutrition and health—and have witnessed a steady increase in obesity, in adult disorders afflicting children and in unexplained cancers. The answer to the question, "How did this happen?" was not easy for me to accept. I had to let go of much of what I thought I knew about nutrition, exercise and public health policy. I had to open my mind to some old and new ideas.

The good news is that Mary and I discovered that the story of our lives did not have to follow the modern script. Even better was the news that you don't have to be an expert to change your life and improve your health. We did just that, losing a combined two hundred-plus pounds without doctors, drugs, dieting or surgery. The best news of all was that losing weight was just the beginning of a physical and mental transformation, one that changed the way we saw the world and ourselves.

But before I tell you about how we changed the direction of our future, I have to tell you how we put the breaks on our past. The amazing fact is that I owe this life-changing experience, this personal reclamation, to an order of take-out chicken.

Part Three
The Road Home

Chapter Eight

An Epiphany and a Plate of Chicken

How could something as simple as a take-out order of chicken save a man's life?

For the first five months of 2003, I was on a temporary work assignment in New York City. I lived out of a suitcase in Manhattan during the week, returning home to Virginia on the weekends. I found myself under considerable stress, and all my meals, five days a week, came from restaurants or through room service. In between meals, I snacked on whatever was available.

My weight, already at a level that would have landed me a position with a traveling circus, then rocketed into the fatosphere. I suffered the usual obesity-related ills: back and joint pain, difficulty walking, shortness of breath, headaches and fatigue. My daily intake of food fluctuated between five thousand and seven thousand calories. In New York, finding a place to eat is never a problem. Add work-related stress, calorie-dense foods and the huge portions served in most restaurants, and maintaining a monumental calorie count is really quite easy. In addition, I drank gallons of fructose-laced soda at twenty-five cents a can and launched nightly raids on the snack bar in my hotel room. I was a walking cautionary tale on the vice of gluttony, an accidental Frankenstein's monster cobbled together from the rubbish heap of processed convenience foods and dietary ignorance.

I realized my diet was a key factor in my declining health, so one day I decided to go on a twenty-four-hour fast. I was only partly successful, as the familiar craving to eat, heightened by a series of Pavlovian triggers, drove me to break my vow and grab some dinner. I found myself at my favorite carry-out deli in lower Manhattan, a little place with the unusual name of The Lord's Deli. I wanted something light, a salad maybe, but the menu mostly featured greasy-looking pasta dishes, so there was little to choose from. Even the pan of sautéed vegetables came smothered in oil. I finally chose a small portion of roasted, skinless chicken breast, accompanied by vegetables I planned to rescue from their hot oil bath once I returned to my hotel room. The chicken, infused with herbs and tasting of butter, was delicious. That night, I drank water with my meal instead of soda and fell into a restless sleep.

The next morning, I felt better than I had in weeks. I had a light breakfast and skipped lunch, saving myself for a repeat of that heavenly chicken. I ordered it again the second night, two pieces this time, and skipped the veggies. The next morning, I was beginning to feel like a changed man. When I walked to work, my back pain was nearly gone. I found that I had more energy and even my normally sour disposition had improved—approaching something that could be described as "sunny." This was all good news, but I couldn't see myself eating nothing but roast chicken for the rest of my life.

It was at that point that I had my epiphany. What if the changes I was experiencing had more to do with what I was NOT eating? For two days I had consumed no glutamates, no cyclamates, no nitrates, no sugar, no soy products, no refined carbohydrates—in short, no processed food.

A REVELATION ON THE HOME FRONT

Two hundred miles away in Virginia, Mary was having a similar revelation. She had received a phone call from her sister, Kathy, with news of an uncle's death. As they were exchanging goodbyes, Kathy remarked on how good she and her husband had been feeling lately. She talked about how they had lost weight and had a surplus of energy. Hungry for some good news, Mary asked her what was it they were doing.

"We're just eating the food we ate when we were young, Mary," came her reply. She continued, "We stopped eating all that processed food." There was a pause. "We eat eggs, Mary, and butter, too."

"Butter? Eggs!" Mary was in shock.

"Don't be afraid of eggs," Kathy said, "They're good for you."

Their conversation continued a bit longer, with Kathy providing the titles of some books she had been reading. Mary listened in fascination. It seemed too good to be true. She quietly dropped the receiver into its cradle and for a moment sat with her hand resting on the phone. Then, her mind made up, she called both of our daughters.

She spoke to them like an officer addressing his troops. "Girls, things are going to be different from now on. The first thing we're going to do is get rid of all this junk food we have in the house. We're going to start cooking our own food. . . ." she paused, gathering her courage, "and we won't be ordering any more pizza—and there won't be any more soda either. We're going to start eating normal. . . ." she groped for the right words, "regular food, like I used to eat when I was a little girl."

The girls exchanged alarmed glances. This sounded serious. Mary went on to explain her decision, as best she could. She had that dead-serious, determined look on her face which meant there was no room for negotiation.

And so commenced what came to be known as "the purge." With trash bags in hand, any food item that failed to pass the test for authenticity was snatched up and consigned to the trash. The authenticity test was quite simple: if an article of food contained ingredients that required a laboratory and people with advanced degrees in chemistry to replicate, it failed.

I called Mary a couple of days later to tell her how much better I felt and was surprised—delighted—to hear that she had come to a similar conclusion.

On the first of June, 2003, we embarked on what would become a "whole foods" way of eating. I had dieted before. I knew the chance of failure was very high, so I decided to do something different this time. Let me say that again, because that moment of clarity represented a turning my life: "I decided to do something different this time."

Albert Einstein said, "The definition of insanity is doing the same thing over and over again and expecting different results." For over a decade, I had followed the same course of action: adopting a new diet, sticking with it for a time before collapsing into my old habits, then regaining any weight I had lost, plus a few bonus pounds for good measure. In every case, I had faithfully followed the rules, resulting in a little success in some cases and a lot of success in others, but the end result was always the same: failure. I realized that in every case, I actually had very little understanding of why the diet worked or didn't work, had no idea of how the human body metabolizes food. I was simply doing what I'd been told by the dietary experts: "Eat a balanced diet and get plenty of exercise." The problem with this advice was that it had never worked for me. I mean, if I knew what a balanced diet was and could stick to it, I would not have had a weight problem to begin with.

I decided I would not commit the crime of "just following orders," as I had done so often before. This time I was going to find the answers for myself. If a whole foods diet really worked, I wanted to know why. I wanted to see the studies that proved it, to uncover the metabolic processes behind it. So I began to read, and as I read I discovered just how wrong-headed America's nutrition policy really is. I came to see why my doctor had never been able to give me any useful advice when it came to weight loss.

I plunged into the history of nutrition politics in America and came up reeling. I read *Food Politics* and *Safe Food* by Marion Nestle, *Fast Food Nation* by Eric Schlosser, *Fat Land* by Greg Critser, the *New York Times* article "What if it's All Been a Big Fat Lie" by Gary Taub, and many other articles, position papers and medical research reports. I looked to science for relief and found that in this area, too, human pride, prejudice and greed had created the flawed dietary policy that millions of Americans now follow. I began to see, for the first time, the folly of a medical industry that expends immense resources on the treatment of obesity-related symptoms, but adopts a hands-off approach when it comes to treating the source of those symptoms: poor nutrition.

Chapter Eight: An Epiphany and a Plate of Chicken

. . . .

I marveled at the zealous adherence to the religion of lowfat eating in the face of clear evidence that for most people this approach does not work. I saw manipulation by powerful industry groups that influenced what my family and I ate and learned how corporations subvert parental authority—by spending millions on sophisticated advertising campaigns in an aggressive effort to market junk food directly to our children through television and in the schools. I saw how this influence is exerted on the people we look to for leadership, from doctors corrupted by pharmaceutical industry largesse to ethically conflicted scientists, politicians and bureaucrats. I saw how economics has played a critical role in shaping nutrition policy. . . and in misshaping us.

In time I came to realize that the mantra of "personal responsibility," intoned by representatives of the food industry and their friends in government is critical to success, but not in the way they intend it. Real personal responsibility means looking past the dogma promulgated by industry interests for their own benefit. As a practical matter, it means learning about basic human physiology and the mechanics of food metabolism. It means adopting an unapologetically discriminatory mind set when it comes to deciding what you put into your body. It means skipping the marketing hype on the front of food packages and reading the ingredient labels on the back. It means learning to identify industry-influenced "journalism" masquerading as unbiased health and nutrition reporting. It means acquiring the language of the scientist to decipher the double-speak and disinformation often employed to hide the real results of industry-sponsored studies on health and nutrition issues.

In my journey, I've discovered that the one-size-fits-all model for diet and nutrition advice does not work for me and does not work for most. I learned that focusing on just one food group is a mistake; that the experts really don't know as much as I thought they did and that they are not telling me everything they do know. I realized that I needed to question all that I knew, or thought I knew, about nutrition.

TIME FOR A CHANGE

In June of 2003, I returned home to Northern Virginia and my family for good. My work on the New York project was over. I took this as a positive sign that it was finally time to make a real change. In the span of just one week, my change in diet from processed to whole foods had already worked a miracle. Suddenly, I had more energy and optimism. I was no longer just plowing through my day, trying to make it through to late-night TV. I had a purpose now, and each new day provided an opportunity to make progress. Where did all this optimism come from?

I realized my diet had weighed me down in ways that I had not expected. When you think about it, though, it shouldn't come as a surprise that food exerts a mental and emotional effect, as well as a physical one. That effect can be a burden or a blessing. Our bodies are just chemical factories, after all. It was a good thing I had so much optimism, because I would need every bit I could muster.

Now for the details of how we got started on our journey and how we stayed the course.

Chapter Nine

The Road Home
Coming back from the brink of oblivion

The buzz of the alarm clock roused me out of a shallow sleep and left me blinking in the dark. I had awakened a half hour earlier and spent the previous thirty minutes moving gently between my dreams and the waking world. I pulled off the covers and in one motion swung toward the side of the bed until I was sitting upright with my feet planted on the floor. Mary stirred in the dark. Two months earlier, moving to an upright position so quickly would have set my head spinning. I would have spent several seconds in a daze, trying to figure out where I was and what I was supposed to do next. But that was two months ago.

Now, in the first week of August 2003, I was instantly awake and alert. The dimly glowing numbers on the alarm clock indicated it was almost four-thirty in the morning. Time to get up. I went to my closet and dressed quickly—gym shorts, a light shirt, athletic socks and running shoes, was all I needed. Muffled footsteps followed by a sliver of light that peeked beneath my closet door announced Mary's intention to join me.

I went downstairs and waited. Mary followed soon after. I retrieved a house key and we both stepped quietly through the darkened lower level of our house to the front door. The street was deserted, but we could hear a chorus of night creatures—frogs, bats, crickets and one insomniac dog, barking somewhere in the dark.

Mary and I walked quietly down the driveway to the street. "Look at these slackers," I said, glancing around at the darkened homes of my neighbors who had the good sense to remain in bed at such an early hour. Mary smiled politely at the tired joke. I had said it every morning for the last two months. We turned south and began the one-mile loop around our neighborhood. The route includes a steep hill that always left me huffing heavily by the time I reached the top. We would walk this route five times on this morning, for more than an hour. It would be the fourth time this week.

This had been our morning ritual for the last few weeks. Up at four-fifteen, out by four-thirty. We had a hard time describing exactly what it was we had been doing for the last two months. We didn't like the word "diet" because it was an inadequate description of the change we had experienced. This was no diet, no temporary adjustment of what we were eating so we could lose a few pounds. We were literally trying to remake ourselves—physically, mentally, emotionally, intellectually and spiritually.

When we started in June, I was unable to do much walking. My back and legs hurt and my hands and feet would swell up uncomfortably, so initially we just changed our diet. I felt better immediately, but for the first two months or so, I saw little weight loss, although my clothes did get looser.

These early morning walks began as simple exercise, but evolved over time into our mobile office, psychiatrist's couch and relationship counseling sessions. Like any couple married for seventeen years, there was much that went unsaid between us. When you walk in circles in the dark for an hour, then two hours, you've got to do something to fill the time, so we talked about life, love, regrets and joys, anger and forgiveness, politics and prose, death and resurrection, our plans, our aspirations and our fears. We talked about anything and everything. It eventually dawned on us that we were getting up early in the morning not to walk, but to enjoy each other's company, discuss the day ahead, plan for our future, laugh, get angry with each other and simply communicate. After more than one year of walking, not only did we grow slimmer, we also grew closer.

Chapter Nine: The Road Home

. . . .

Later, as we grew healthier—and were able to see a future for ourselves that transcended the confining roles defined by an over-commercialized society—we exercised our entrepreneurial muscles and worked up the courage to pursue business opportunities we had only dreamed of before. Our morning walks, which previously had revolved around our personal lives, now doubled as business meetings. Our one-mile course became our new conference room.

It wasn't always easy. Sometimes we would finish a walk in silence, with a bruised ego or an aching heart. Other times, we laughed over some nearly-forgotten incident until tears welled up in our eyes. Usually, however, our walks were a joyous celebration of the new future we envisioned together—a future without the discomfort of poor health. I was amazed at how, after so many years together, so much had been left unsaid between us and so much was left to say.

Our daughters slept during these early morning expeditions, but by the time they awoke, the house was filled with the aroma of breakfast. On most days breakfast included eggs—real eggs, not the anemic egg whites that I had subsisted on during my lowfat days. The eggs were often accompanied by nitrate-free bacon or done up as an omelet with vegetables and meat left over from yesterday's dinner. Sometimes we had unhomogenized whole milk with our breakfast.

MORE CHANGES

Besides our early morning walks, the most obvious change in our household was the food we ate. Gone were the frozen bags of pre-cooked chicken from the bulk foods warehouse. The thick slabs of frozen heat-and-serve toast that we used to eat were missing too, and there were no more empty bags of chips, bottles of soda, or take-out pizza boxes to gather up for the weekly trash collection. The drive-thru cashiers at several of the fast food outlets I frequented were, no doubt, concerned over my absence, as I am certain I contributed significantly to their monthly revenue goals.

We did most of our shopping at the local farmers' market and at stores that specialized in whole foods products. We tried to stick to the basics: meat, seafood, fruits, vegetables and dairy products. Of course, our parting of the ways with processed food could best be described as a separation rather than a full-fledged divorce. At the time, I still believed that soy was a healthy food for me and continued to purchase tofu products. I was not yet completely immune to the lure of junk food either.

THE LOW POINT

One day after work, I had to stop for gas. I was hungry and wanted something to eat for the ninety-minute commute. I surveyed the gas station store aisles and found nothing but snack foods. I don't even remember what my excuse was, but somehow, I rationalized the purchase of a family-sized bag of potato chips as a "healthy" alternative to the rest of the fare available. I gassed up and kept one eye on the interstate while I struggled to open the bag of chips with one hand.

There's an old movie, *The Days of Wine and Roses*, which stars Jack Lemon as an alcoholic struggling to overcome his demons. In one riveting scene, Jack's character attempts to rehabilitate himself by spending time with his father-in-law, helping out with the family's garden business. Jack had hidden a bottle of liquor in one of the potted plants in the greenhouse and had planned to sneak in at night and drink it while everyone else was asleep. Unfortunately, he forgot which planter he hid the bottle in. What started as a simple recovery operation turned into a manic search-and-destroy mission instead. By the time he found the bottle, he had completely destroyed the greenhouse. He then got drunk, which only made him feel worse.

I plowed into that bag of greasy, salty, artificially flavored potato chips like the drunk in *The Days of Wine and Roses*. I told myself, "I'll only eat a few," just enough to take the edge off my hunger, but I knew I would not—could not—stop. When it was over, I crumpled up the empty bag with my greasy free hand and flung it to the floor of the car in disgust. I had managed to stay "clean" for several weeks and now this. What's worse, my hunger had not abated. I just felt sick, physically and emotionally. It was then that I saw so clearly the control that unhealthy food had over me.

Chapter Nine: The Road Home

It made me angry at myself and at the nameless, faceless corporate entity that made access to these foods so easy and inviting—like the friendly neighborhood drug dealer who always has just what you think you need. That was my low point. I would never reach that point again.

FOOD TRACKER

Early hunter-gatherer societies had to be skilled at tracking their food if they wanted to eat. In September of 2003, I too learned to track my food. I acquired a new weapon in my arsenal of weight loss gadgets, a software program called "Diet and Exercise." I installed it on the Palm handheld that I took with me everywhere. This program enabled me accurately to track the food I ate, along with the number of calories and the macronutrient breakdown. For a month prior to purchasing the software, I had kept a written account, noting every morsel that passed my lips. At the end of the day, I would enter this data into a spreadsheet. It was a cumbersome but effective way to track my food intake.

The electronic tracker was wonderful because it had a huge database of foods and enabled me to run "what-if" scenarios. If I was trying to stick to a set number of calories on a given day, I could plug in different meal options to determine how much of a particular food item I could consume without exceeding my calorie count. My daily calorie intake averaged around two thousand. This number was important, because as someone who had paid little attention to how much I ate for the past ten years, I needed to relearn how to control my portions. Doing so helped teach my body to adjust to fewer calories, although it was only through eating whole, satisfying foods that I was able to control my portions.

Another benefit of food tracking was that when I reviewed what I had eaten over the course of a month, I could see patterns in my eating behavior that I might not otherwise have noticed. I saw, for instance, that I ate more on Saturdays than any other day of the week. I also noted that when I tried to cut my calories below what was a normal amount for me (about two thousand), I could only maintain this reduced-calorie level for two or three days. After that, my records typically revealed a sudden spike in food intake, a binge, usually on the third or fourth day. I could also see connections between food intake and mood. If I was stuck in traffic on the way home, there was usually a spike in calorie consumption soon afterward. This information was very helpful because it made me more aware—not just of what I was eating, but when I was eating and why. Thus, having identified harmful behavior patterns, I was able to work on changing them.

I was sold on the value of food tracking, but Mary hated it. Attending to the minutia of tracking ran counter to the more freestyle approach she took to cooking and eating. She had far more control than I over her eating behavior and did not need the extra help that tracking provides. Inevitably, we locked horns over the issue. A typical pre-dinner conversation went something like this:

"Mmmm, that smells good. Are we having chili?" I'd ask.

"Yes," would come her clipped reply, along with a sudden drop in temperature in the room.

I'd start with a little small talk and work toward my real point of interest. "I didn't eat much for lunch and traffic was pretty bad today. I've really been looking forward to dinner." I'd pause to gauge her response, and then continue. "Hey, are those jalapeño peppers I smell? Oh yeah, you're making it spicy the way I like it—so what else is in there?" This was the moment of truth.

She would take a deep breath, set her jaw, then list the ingredients without taking her eyes off the stove or stopping what she was doing. "Hamburger, peppers, onions, tomatoes. . . ." The list continued until she was finished and then silence.

"So how much hamburger did you put in?"

A long silence. When she cooked, Mary made do with whatever ingredients were available—a pinch here, a smidgen there. That was her style. As mother, home school teacher, primary cook, soccer practice chauffeur, household accountant and hair braider, she found food and ingredient tracking an unnecessary complication to her already busy life. Her reply usually came in the form of a rough estimate which I generally regarded as an inadequate reply to my demand for excruciating exactness. These opening shots served as a preamble to an undeclared cold war expressed through exasperated sighs, cold shoulders, steely glares and stony silence. Thankfully, this was the only issue we ever clashed over as we worked toward remaking our lives.

THE HOLIDAYS: A DIETER'S NIGHTMARE

By October of 2003, I was feeling like a new man. Four months of healthier eating and exercise had worked a miracle. I was tracking my weight and was overjoyed to see that I had lost almost six pounds per week for several weeks. My clothes were falling off me and my energy was up. I no longer minded going walking at four-thirty in the morning. In fact, I looked forward to it. Along with rising early, I had finally adjusted to going to bed at nine o'clock in the evening. Giving up late night TV was the only way to ensure I could get enough sleep to keep such early hours. Although my weight still hovered northwards of three hundred pounds, I had lost about fifty pounds and I felt great. My goal for the year was to break the three hundred-pound barrier by Christmas.

Anyone who has ever tried to lose weight knows that the holidays are a treacherous time of year. From about mid-October through the end of December, food becomes a principal component of every thought, conversation and action. It starts with Halloween candy, complete with orange and black sugary confections, candied apples and those styrofoam-like peanut candies.

Next comes the Mount Everest of food holidays: Thanksgiving. When I was growing up, the days leading up to turkey day turned my every-day world into a mythical land of candied ham, sweet potato pies, banana pudding, spicy dressing with succulent chunks of meat and crunchy celery, potato salad with sweet nuggets of apples, oven-baked rolls smothered in butter, cornbread and collard greens, sweet onions, cranberry sauce and homemade ice cream.

Finally, Christmas. Another turkey, ham or both. Cookies, cheese and caramel popcorn, more pies, hard candies, mounds of salted mixed nuts, sweet apples, oranges and tangerines and a cake or two. Even though in my adult years we had scaled back the amount of holiday food we ate, it was still the food season as far as I was concerned.

At Christmas, the strong are separated from the weak. In the old days, we would have given in to the temptations of the holidays, packing in more food and packing on more weight, but not this time. Our mostly whole foods diet had an unexpected effect on us. Whenever we attempted to lose weight in the past, it was always a struggle. We were always shadowed by cravings for the sticky-sweet salty foods we loved, so we were a bit surprised to find that those cravings had evaporated.

This was a revelation. We were beginning to understand that our carbohydrate-rich, nutrient-poor, processed-food diet actually made us want to eat more, sparking cravings for certain foods that always defeated us in the end. We decided not to buy any Halloween candy, but Thanksgiving and Christmas turned out to be quite a surprise when we discovered on December thirty-first, 2003 that we actually lost weight over the holidays. I did not cross the three hundred-pound barrier as I had hoped, but I was much closer.

THE WESTON A. PRICE FOUNDATION

It was in December of 2003 that I discovered the Weston A. Price Foundation, an organization dedicated to the research of Dr. Price, which educates consumers about the value of nutrient-dense food and traditional diets—and helps them find these foods.

Dr. Price's work and that of the Foundation affected me deeply, in part because it made so much sense and answered a lot of questions. The chief message of the Foundation was that food had to provide liberal amounts of the nutrients the body needs—not the minimal Recommended Daily Allowances, but *liberal* amounts. Otherwise physical degeneration will occur, with each generation becoming less fit than the one before.

Finally . . . here was a plausible explanation for my family's decline in health with each succeeding generation. I could see now why, despite my best efforts to exercise and eat right, I still gained weight. And here was an explanation for the increase in overweight grade-school-aged kids.

I was beginning to see why exercise never seemed to provide the return on investment that I thought it should. It was becoming clear to me just how critical a role food played in my health. I never believed the argument—popular with sectors of the food industry and many health officials—that it didn't matter what I ate so long as I exercised. I didn't believe the subtle message from many of the experts that obesity is simply the result of laziness and a conscious choice to overeat. I knew I wasn't lazy, and I knew that I never chose to be fat. I knew that some foods did make me feel lazy sometimes while other foods gave me energy. The premise of the diet professionals, that all food is the same, just didn't match my experience.

Also, it didn't make sense to me that good health was defined by body weight and nothing else. I knew a number of people, such as diabetics, who were very thin, but being thin didn't make them healthy. But this was the message I had been hearing for most of my life: health equals thin and thin equals a lowfat diet.

By focusing only on calories, nutrition leaders and industry interests had engaged in a calculated effort to avoid any discussion about the nutritive quality of our food. And since fats have twice as many calories as protein or carbohydrates, these experts argued that the ticket to good health was a scale-back of fat to the bare minimum—no egg yolks, no cream, no fat on your meat, no lard and no butter.

Yet Weston Price discovered that these fats carry the most important vitamins of all.

When I was a kid, no one counted calories. We simply ate the food that was available. A lot of this food—full-fat dairy products and red meat—were the very things I had been warned to avoid for most of my adult life. How was it possible, then, that once people became more conscious about diet and weight, started counting calories and eating diet food, the percentage of overweight and obese people increased so quickly?

Something was seriously wrong with what I came to see as the Fat Hypothesis. It seemed the lowfat, high-carbohydrate, processed food prescription for preventing obesity and heart disease was actually causing these epidemics.

The other reason the work of Dr. Price and the Foundation struck a chord with me is that so much of what they taught sounded like my mother's advice. She never badgered me to go outside and get exercise. She didn't have to. I was a pretty active kid. She did, however, spend a lot of time extolling the healthful virtues of traditional foods. She would have been appalled at my consumption of simulated soy foods, breakfast pastries, margarine and fast food. For most of my childhood, she always kept a garden in our backyard. She believed in the concept of organic produce long before the idea became mainstream. She purchased a side of beef once and in the good times always kept our freezer well stocked with everything from filet mignon to stew bones. She knew how to render lard from fatback and understood the nutritive value of soup made from bones or fish heads. She plied me with chicken soup and bone broth when I was ill and gave me cod liver oil to keep me well. She believed in cooking from scratch and rarely bought food pre-cooked. She was wary of food additives.

Mother was a voracious consumer of books on health. And yet, despite her commitment to good health, she was not immune to the seductive temptation of affordable convenience foods. For a time, she strayed from her roots, but eventually returned to the food she knew best. At the age of forty-three years I discovered what most of us discover eventually. Mom was right all along.

THERE'S NO PLACE LIKE HOME, FOR EXERCISE

In September we decided, as an early Christmas gift, to convert an unfinished room in our basement into a home gym. We already had a flat weight bench, a rowing machine and an older treadmill, but this equipment was crowded into a small space. There wasn't really enough room for everything, so we kept the treadmill folded up and moved the rowing machine from its storage space when we wanted to use it. The lack of space often gave me an excuse not to exercise, so when we decided to turn the spare room into a gym, it seemed like the perfect solution.

First we brought in workmen to hang the drywall and apply the paint. We took over from there. I laid down a padded floor made of interlocking pieces of dense black foam, then ran a four-inch black strip around the entire room to create the effect of a baseboard. Next we hung three large mirrors along one wall, transforming the once-drab room into something that looked like a gym. Last, we brought in the equipment which included the treadmill, the flat bench, a set of dumbbells and a barbell bench with stations for bench pressing, butterflies, leg presses and preacher curls. We also put in a stationary bike and, later, a new treadmill, an elliptical machine and a heavy bag for boxing. As a finishing touch, I added a black locker where we stored our weight-lifting equipment, boxing gloves and towels. A large industrial fan and a CD stereo system completed the furnishings. It was good, but the walls were too bare, so I added a white board for writing out the day's exercise routine and a stainless steel peg board for posting pictures or notes on the wall. We decided not to install a television as we thought it might be a distraction—and a temptation to return to our old ways.

When I walked into the gym and closed the door, an amazing thing happened. Suddenly, I wasn't at home anymore. I was at the gym. I found that by creating a total exercise-immersion environment, I was motivated to do just that. I realize a home gym isn't an option for everyone, but when I consider what a difference it has made in my life, I will never be without one again. For me, spare bedrooms, game rooms and home theatres all take a back seat in priority to a home gym.

I enjoy exercising, but I still believe it has been oversold as a cure-all for everything. Why, for instance, is it so difficult to stick to a routine? Why does something that is supposed to be so healthy hurt so much? Like many things in life, exercise has two faces. The right amount of sensible exercise, supported with good nutrition, can be a boon to your health. Too much of the wrong exercise on the wrong diet can do the opposite. Let's take a look at the myth of exercise and explore ways to make exercise work for you.

Chapter Ten

What You Don't Know About Exercise
Why exercise alone won't solve your health problems

The new dietary guidelines for Americans recommend that those adults on weight-loss programs should engage in sixty to ninety minutes of moderate intensity exercise each day. The diet doctors never tire of reminding us that the key to weight loss is simple: eat less, exercise more. Some experts will go so far as to suggest that what you eat is irrelevant, as long as you maintain a caloric expenditure that exceeds your caloric intake. Exercise has been touted as a cure-all for many ailments. With all the hyperbole surrounding the benefits of regular exercise, it's easy to see why many people view it as the magic bullet that can solve all their problems.

There's little doubt that great benefits derive from exercise. Our bodies were designed to be challenged physically. Our muscles revel in the task of straining against opposing forces; running, swimming and sports exhilarate us. Our exquisitely designed cardiovascular system hums merrily along when our demand for blood and oxygen increases during aerobic workouts. And let us not forget the psychological and emotional benefits derived from physical work as well.

Once, when I worked as a software developer, my co-workers and I decided to rearrange our office space by reconfiguring the layout of our cubicles. The individual slabs that made up the cubicle walls were old and quite heavy. As software developers, we normally spent our days comfortably settled in front of a computer. On this day however, we took turns grunting, sweating and cursing as we dragged the huge slabs of cloth-covered metal from one end of the office to the other. Despite the difficulty of the work, the pinched fingers and stubbed toes, I recall feeling elated by the end of the day. It wasn't just the sense of euphoria one experiences from physical labor, it was also the sense of accomplishment and the feeling that I had actually completed something important, a rare experience in the software world. I left work that day feeling like a new man, albeit a sweaty and disheveled one.

So what's wrong with exercise? Nothing. The problem is that exercise has been grossly oversold as a cure-all for weight loss and health maintenance. Take the new guidelines for example. If you're overweight, it's very likely that you're also out of shape. Exercising sixty to ninety minutes a day is a noble goal, but it may not be possible for you in your condition. If the only way for you to lose weight is by exercising for an hour and a half each day, you're stuck in a catch-22 scenario. This is a perfect example of weight-loss theory colliding with weight-gain reality. The exercise myth holds that exercise alone provides the answer to losing weight, maintaining weight loss, and sustaining a high level of fitness.

Anyone who has ever started a new year by joining a gym and spending the next two weeks working feverishly to get in shape eventually experiences the down-side of exercise. After punishing the body for days on end, you invariably fall ill from overexertion or wind up injuring yourself.

Of course, you could always take it slow by adopting the familiar "small steps" approach that we've heard so much about recently. Small steps may work for someone who is relatively fit already, but for those of us who are grossly overweight, small steps simply won't work for the same reason that trying to fill an empty swimming pool one teacup at a time won't work. While it is technically feasible, it's not very likely to result in success. The small-steps approach to weight loss suffers from the assumption that you can solve a big problem with little effort and change your behavior toward exercise without changing anything else in your life.

. . . .

It's simply not realistic to think that walking a few extra steps per day is sufficient to counter the damage wrought by years of inactivity and a diet that consists of bagels and donuts for breakfast, chicken nuggets, burgers and fries for lunch, and a bucket of spaghetti and meatballs for dinner. Real success in weight loss and real health gains come from developing a strategic multidisciplinary plan that incorporates the following steps:

- A willingness to educate yourself about how your body works;
- A willingness to make a lifelong commitment toward your goals;
- Soliciting support from family, friends and professionals;
- Creating harmony in your life by identifying areas of stress and working toward solutions to reduce that stress;
- Cutting through the hype of our over-commercialized consumer society and learning to identify what really is important in your life;
- Adopting an improved approach to what you eat, with an emphasis on real foods;
- Developing and implementing a realistic exercise program;
- Getting good sleep;
- Applying your newfound sense of empowerment toward achieving personal goals;
- Sharing what you've learned with others.

I have found that any weight-loss effort that omits anything on this list is doomed to failure. It may be possible to lose weight and appear healthy through sheer willpower and an above average tolerance for pain. Over time, however, our bodies will simply break down under the twin burdens of too much exercise and too little nutrition. Take a look at marathon runners toward the end of the pack as they cross the finish line. These are high-performance athletes, yet exercise can turn them into stumbling corpses.

Many weight-loss plans call for restricted calories based on lowfat, low-energy foods. This is the reduced-calorie side of the diet equation. Imagine eating lots of fiber-rich salad, a sliver of skinless chicken breast and drinking lots of water. Full? Of course you are. Satisfied? Not likely. Now go exercise. According to some of the most popular weight loss plans, you're now expected to go out and engage in moderate intensity exercise for sixty to ninety minutes, and you're expected to do this over and over again. Good luck.

Do we really believe the Great Plains Indians were fueling up on salads before engaging in the demanding labor of running down buffalo? Were the Inuit of Alaska topping off their tanks with lowfat meal replacement shakes before heading out across the ice to track seal?

When I tried to exercise and follow a lowfat diet plan, I found I usually grew tired long before an hour was up. Very often, by the last fifteen minutes of exercise, my workouts looked like the thrashings of a dying man. I had used up most of the "energy" from my meager diet in the first fifteen to twenty minutes. I usually felt like a failure at the end of one of these sessions. Imagine having a full stomach, but still feeling hungry, and now, because of a poor workout, add mild depression to this stew of troubles. Try repeating this scenario over the course of a couple weeks. It's easy to see why people simply give up, order an extra large pizza and plant themselves in front of the TV. The idea that you can consume less energy at the table but somehow expend more energy in the gym is ridiculous. While it is true that burning more calories than you consume will result in weight loss, this premise is only true if you've consumed enough of the right kind of energy to fuel both your body and your mind. Failing this, your workouts may only serve to remind you of how miserable you are. The high failure rate that many of us experience when it comes to dieting and exercise suggests that low-energy eating coupled with attempts at high-energy exercise fail far more often than they succeed. Yet many experts swear by this method. When failure inevitably occurs, the problem is never their flawed method, but *your* apparent lack of willpower.

One of the latest trends in exercise is the ten-thousand-steps fad. Pedometers have been flying off the shelves as people try to meet the new dietary guidelines by walking ten thousand steps per day. This is a noble cause to be sure, but if you're overweight and in poor physical condition, walking ten thousand steps everyday is virtually impossible.

When I weighed over four hundred pounds, walking even one hundred steps was difficult. I found that no amount of willpower could overcome a knee that slips out of place and a lower back that grinds with pain after only five minutes of walking. Consuming a low-energy, high-carbohydrate diet based on highly processed foods, grains, salads and vegetable oils, and then trying to exercise for thirty minutes, let alone sixty to ninety, was simply out of the question. My diet at the time left me listless, unsatisfied, fatigued and despondent. Even if I had somehow possessed the physical energy to exercise, I still would have lacked the mental desire to do so. Why, then, has the government devised new dietary and fitness recommendations which, for people like me, are practically guaranteed to fail?

Yet the new dietary guidelines put much more emphasis on physical activity than the previous ones. Why such a focus on exercise? I'll tell you why: the food lobby is very powerful. No one in that industry wants to see restrictions put on the foods that yield the highest profits, namely most of the products on your grocer's shelf, products composed of cheap ingredients—starch, sugar, MSG, trans fats and soy—in other words, processed convenience foods. The dietary guidelines put so much focus on exercise because that allows the creators of the guidelines to avoid the politically sensitive issue of food. The focus on exercise evades the unpleasant task of telling the truth about the food we eat and setting meaningful restrictions on the types of food we consume.

How else can we justify dietary advice that says "there's no such thing as bad food," dietary advice that tells us the quantity of food—the amount of calories it contains—is what's really important, not the quality. In other words, it's OK to eat pretty much anything so long as you count calories. By this reasoning, a diet of soda, glazed donuts and potato chips is acceptable, as long as you don't eat too much and get plenty of exercise. This anything-goes approach is good news for the food industry, but bad news for the rest of us. By putting the focus on exercise, the food industry is absolved of any responsibility for the nation's growing weight problem.

Of course, some of the blame falls on us, as we have become a woefully sedentary people and have refused to educate ourselves about how our bodies work and what we should eat. But sharing responsibility is the foundation of a civilized society. Where, then, is the social responsibility of an industry that makes unsubstantiated health claims about its products, promotes fattening foods for dieters, cloaks harmful additives like MSG under consumer-friendly names like "flavors," and preys on children with empty treats designed to heighten their sensitivity to the very foods that contribute most to poor health?

Where is the social responsibility of our elected officials whom we have trusted to protect us from a predatory free market system that puts corporate profit above personal health? And where is the social responsibility of our prescription-drug-addicted medical community? Why have they wasted decades obsessed about dietary animal fat when they knew, or should have known, that it was liquid and partially hydrogenated vegetable oils in snack foods, baked goods and fried foods that were harming us, and that excessive sugars, starches and additives in America's diet of ready-to-eat convenience foods were major destroyers of our health?

One final myth about exercise is the idea that you can form a new exercise habit in just six months. Occasionally this happens, but not often. Just look at the failure rate of most diets and exercise routines. In many cases, we never make it to the six-month mark. Rarely does exercise become a lifelong habit. I found that after a year of vegetarianism, and then another six months on a low-carb diet combined with regular trips to the gym, quitting was easy. I believe my failure in both cases had everything to do with an inadequate diet. When I finally improved my diet in the summer of 2003, maintaining a routine of regular exercise suddenly became possible. Habits, for the most part, can only be formed when we derive some pleasure from the activity in question. Because I found little pleasure in vegetarianism and spending long hours in a commercial gym, those activities never became habits. If you are on a diet or participating in an exercise program from which you derive little joy, your chance of lasting success is nil.

THE TRUTH ABOUT EXERCISE

So what's the truth about exercise? Exercise is essential for weight loss and good health, but exercise is only one strategy in a multi-part approach to better health. Before you put on your walking shoes, be aware that without a nutrient-dense diet, you're only addressing one part of the problem. Before you assume you know which foods are preventing you from getting the full benefit of exercise, make sure you've read the chapters in Section 4 and reviewed the resources section. It's also important to reduce stress in your life. Getting plenty of sleep on a regular basis is another factor that helped us achieve success in our efforts to lose weight.

WHY IS EXERCISE SO DIFFICULT?

Even with a good diet, reduced stress and plenty of sleep, you may still find regular exercise difficult to sustain. Historically speaking, exercise—that is, the act of engaging in a physically demanding activity for the sole purpose of maintaining physical fitness—is a relatively new concept. Our hunter-gatherer ancestors and their agrarian descendents had little need for exercise. Why would they, given the physically demanding lives they led? Except for professional athletes and others whose work is physically demanding, most of us can manage our daily lives with very little exercise. This is a markedly different situation compared to that of our ancestors, whose very survival required them to be physically active.

If you were to propose to a homesteader of the 1890s that he should get up in the morning and go to a place where he could run on a treadmill and lift heavy objects, he would think you were mad. He would wonder why anyone would waste all that energy running in place and working up a sweat when it could more fruitfully be applied to mending fences, building a barn or hunting for food. The lives we lived were once in balance with our bodies' requirements for optimal health. In our modern lives today, where much of the physical labor has been eliminated, we have fallen out of balance with activity needs.

In my early career as a graphic designer, I often worked at a large drafting table standing up. In the days before computers, I used the familiar tools of the draftsman—the T-square, triangle and ruler. My work required a fair amount of reaching, bending and squatting. In those days, my profession required me to move about the office where I worked. I often spent up to half my day on my feet. Today, I sit in an office in front of a computer. With a telephone, computer, the Internet and email, I can conduct my entire business from my desk. The price I and many others have paid for this "progress" is chronic inactivity and compromised health.

To compensate, we exercise. Make no mistake, this exercise is a substitute for the real work we used to do. The problem is that while our bodies are designed to handle physical challenge, as humans our brains are hard-wired to work only when there is a clear purpose for the work. Without the clear purpose of building shelter, defending our family or finding food, physical exercise can seem irrelevant. This is why walking on a treadmill is a non-productive activity, since even the dullest toddler knows that the purpose of walking is to get from point A to point B. If a man is required to walk five miles each day to tend his flock, he does so because there is a clear purpose in the effort directly connected to his own survival. If the same man attempts to walk on a treadmill for five miles every day, the effort may seem pointless, even when his doctor insists he needs to exercise to protect his heart.

For most of us, no amount of scare mongering about premature death from heart disease, diabetes and stroke is enough to motivate us to exercise regularly. It is only when we have had a close call with the reaper that we finally see the relevant connection to exercise, but even a brush with death loses its sting after a sufficient amount of time has passed and the football-and-spicy-nachos season rolls around again.

The challenge is how to make exercise relevant enough in our lives so that we are motivated to do it on a regular basis. Most of us live in densely packed housing in the city or the suburbs, so wandering out to tend our flock on a daily basis is not an option. If you are fortunate enough to live in a pedestrian-friendly area where walking is feasible, you can leave the car in the garage and walk to the store, the bus stop or even the office. Parking farther from the entrance to your place of business and using the stairs are two "small steps" you can take, but they won't really contribute much to your overall health unless your company has a parking lot the size of Delaware. There's always the option of chucking your modern life, selling your home in the suburbs and moving out to the country on a few acres in order to create a life more conducive to good health. For some people this really is an option, but for most of us it isn't. What should we do then?

WHAT WE DID

Mary and I realized that we couldn't transfer all of the exercise we needed into something other than exercise, but we did discover several ways to make exercise more meaningful. In addition to our morning walks, we added bicycling. We found that riding a bike the ten miles or so to the farmers' market became a highly relevant activity, one connected with procuring food. We live on a half-acre parcel with a large swath of unruly lawn. At least twice a month, Mary pushes a lawn mower up and down the hill at the back of the lot, achieving a workout that rivals anything she can do in the gym.

When we put in a raised-bed garden, we had to purchase fill dirt to fill the two garden boxes we built. More than a half ton of dirt was hauled to our home by the supplier and dumped in the street—thirty yards away from the garden. We spent the entire day hauling wheelbarrow loads of dirt from the street to the garden. When the boxes were filled, we had to haul the extra dirt an additional ten yards up the steep hill behind our house. It was back-breaking work, but it left us exhilarated. These alternate exercise activities were not random "small steps," but were part of a larger plan to add more physical activity to our daily lives.

Everything from turning the earth in our garden to trimming trees and cleaning out the garage became a meaningful opportunity to exercise. If you examine your life closely, you can probably find ways to make exercise more meaningful, too. Of course, once you learn to make some exercises more practical, you may discover that the "impractical" ones, like walking on a treadmill, are easier and more enjoyable.

Of course, we also exercised in our gym. We needed a few weeks with our new eating plan before we had the mental and physical energy to begin our program. And build us up it did. I was actually quite surprised at how much better I felt after only a few weeks away from most of the convenience foods we used to eat.

When we did begin to exercise, I decided that it would be useful for us to keep track of which exercises we did and how often we did them. I created a checklist on the computer that listed several exercises, like walking and weight-lifting routines. I included a row that showed the dates for the month and a column for checking off which days I exercised and which exercise I did on each day. I printed out this chart and stuck it up on the wall in the gym.

We set a goal of five days per week for exercise, alternating aerobic exercise (walking, jogging and the treadmill) with anaerobic exercise like weight lifting.

One final point regarding exercise: do not fall victim to the myth of the perfect body. For women, this means that you should not feel compelled to transform yourself into a life-sized Barbie doll. For men, this means that you shouldn't get stressed over the fact that you don't have washboard abs. These models are part of a consumer engineering effort designed to make us feel bad about ourselves so we'll continue to buy products and services that will supposedly make us happier. They won't. It is important to love the body you have, whatever its imperfections.

THE TOOLS WE USE: FITNESS TRACKERS

I was no stranger to exercise, but when I decided to make a change for the better, I knew I needed something other than just a fuzzy idea in my head about my workout program. I needed a real plan and a way to track my progress. Why track? Early on, I was feeling a bit frustrated because I wanted to see instant results. Two months after I began my exercise program I didn't see much progress. I thought I was working out almost every day—or was I? I checked my tracker, which was a simple printed spreadsheet with a list of exercises, dates and a checkbox to denote when I exercised. I discovered that, most weeks, I was working out only three days a week. That wasn't how I remembered it, of course, but my tracker told the truth.

I also created a spreadsheet for weight training exercises with space for dates, sets and reps. I found lots of professionally produced video clips on the Internet that demonstrated how to do the exercises properly. Whenever I worked out, I simply checked off that day. I found it helpful to alternate exercises so as not to overwork any particular body part, and to alternate workout days and factor in an occasional day off.

BODY FAT ANALYZER

Your body fat is the ratio of fat to lean body mass (muscle). A quick check on the Internet will turn up a body fat chart that shows what your body fat should allegedly be for your weight and height. I don't consider these charts to be the definitive word on what my body fat ratio should be. Remember, one-size-fits-all solutions rarely work, but they can provide a helpful guide.

You can measure your body fat in a number of ways. I use an impedance device, an electronic device with metal sensors that send a low-level electrical signal through your body. No, it doesn't hurt. The lean tissue in your body has a higher percentage of water and so conducts the signal more quickly than does the fat in your body. The device then calculates your body fat with these data.

So how accurate is this method? I don't know. Depending upon the device used, what time of day you do the measurement, and whether you've recently drunk any water, you can get different results. So why use it? When I was a vegetarian, I lost about fifty pounds, but I ended up weak and I tired easily. I suspect that along with the fat, I lost quite a bit of muscle mass as well. Measuring my body fat, even if the measurement is inaccurate, is useful for showing whether I'm losing fat or gaining muscle mass over time. I perform the measurement at the same time of day under the same conditions so the results are consistent. I found this to be a useful tool for tracking progress.

Mary doesn't share my obsession with technology and my penchant for gathering arcane bits of data, and so she does not bother checking her body fat. "I can see all the body fat I want in a mirror, thank you," is her characteristic comment.

BATHROOM SCALES

Some of you may be afraid of the scale. I know I was. Get over it. It's not like people haven't noticed that you have a weight problem. The irony is that the only person you're keeping this "secret" from is you. It's natural to want to avoid bad news, but avoiding a problem prevents you from solving it, so get thee to a scale and face the fat. Can't find a scale at the local discount-mart that goes up high enough? You may need to order one. I've seen scales that measure up to four hundred pounds. I've read about scales that go higher.

My scale is an analog scale, the kind with the red needle. Personally I don't trust the electronic ones since, if I stood on my laptop, I wouldn't expect it to work properly either. This is my own personal bias, as I've heard there's not much difference between an electronic and an analog scale.

Use the scale, but do not live and die by it. One of the unsolved mysteries of weight loss is the fact that you can drop clothing sizes, look slimmer in the mirror, and elicit envious stares from strangers, yet still weigh the same for many weeks in a row. The explanation typically offered is that you're gaining muscle as you're losing fat, and that's how you're able to become physically smaller but weigh the same. I don't completely buy this argument, as it would have to be some kind of coincidence for you to gain in muscle the exact amount of fat lost, and unless you're a high-performance athlete, don't expect to gain a lot of muscle anyway. Use the scale as just one measure of your success, a guide, nothing more. How often you weigh yourself is up to you: once a week, once a day, or once a month, it's your call.

TAPE MEASURE

Bathroom scales can be frustrating when they fail to register obvious progress evidenced by your clothes. A tape measure may be just the ticket for helping you see your success. Common body parts to measure are the waist, hips, thigh, chest, neck and calf.

For some people, finding your waist may represent a challenge. Unfortunately, fitness experts can't seem to agree on where exactly the waist is. Some say above the navel. Some say below the navel. Others say just below the rib cage, or the thinnest section of your lower trunk. What do you do if there is no "thinnest" section of your trunk, or your rib cage has gone missing? I shoot for the area between the navel and the rib cage. Close enough, I think.

BLOOD PRESSURE GAUGE

If you're overweight, your blood pressure is probably higher than recommended. There are different schools of thought on what this means. Some medical experts believe that hypertension is a precursor to heart disease while others believe that heart disease comes first, and that high blood pressure is symptomatic of an ill heart. Confused? Here's more to baffle you: the numbers that indicate high blood pressure have been revised downward over the years. One hundred twenty over eighty used to be considered a normal blood pressure, but this number has recently been redefined as "pre-hypertensive." Some observers suggest that this change in the guidelines has little to do with concern for our health and everything to do with expanding the market for expensive blood pressure medications. I tend to agree. Whatever side of the argument you fall on, you should research the whole story on blood pressure, then make your own decisions. Exercise, a good diet and weight loss have been shown to improve blood pressure. Just remember that blood pressure goes up naturally and gradually with age (the old standard was your age plus one hundred over ninety). Some people can even go off their medication by controlling their blood pressure through lifestyle changes. We did.

FITNESS EQUIPMENT FOR THE GYM

A set of dumbbells and a weight bench is one of the cheapest, most versatile and most effective investments you can make. There are literally hundreds of exercises you can do with dumbbells and a bench (an incline bench is even better). It goes without saying that heavy objects made of iron can be dangerous when used improperly. Study up first, start slow and be safe.

I also recommend a barbell bench that allows for bench presses, preacher curls, leg lifts, etc. When I'm walking outside, I sometimes use a weight vest and ankle weights. Walking with weights can be a good low-impact way to increase the intensity of your walks. Weight vests can be adjusted from zero up to their maximum weight and can feel quite heavy when you first try one on. If you use a vest, make sure you're already in fairly good shape. Start small, real small, with very light weights (five to ten pounds). Go slow, be safe.

Even though I am a big proponent of home gyms, commercial gyms can still be a very valuable component in your exercise plan. In fact, from time to time, I'll sign up for a month's membership with a local gym, just so I can utilize different equipment and experience greater diversity in my exercise routines.

AEROBICS

I break a sweat with a stationary gym bike. I use an elliptical machine in my gym and prefer to do my running on a treadmill, since it absorbs the shock of running much better than asphalt, which can be brutal on the legs, feet and joints. If you do buy home gym equipment, it's worth saving up for sturdier equipment that can take a pounding. The cheap stuff is a poor investment in the long run. Get some opinions and feedback from friends who exercise or from the most knowledgeable person you can find at your local gym.

Another useful workout tool is a rebounder. A rebounder is a mini-trampoline that lets you work up a sweat safely, and it can be fun, too. Your workout on a rebounder can be as low-impact as you like. If you fatigue easily, this might be a good option for you.

For real fun, I like to work out on my heavy punching bag. I use lightweight boxing gloves or my fingerless weight-lifting gloves. There's nothing like the satisfaction of hammering that bag and imagining yourself in a match with an annoying co-worker. To heighten the fantasy, I listen to a custom CD I made with a music soundtrack, crowd noises and an announcer. The background music, a driving bass-beat that's perfect for boxing, is set to loop every two minutes so I can do two-minute rounds. One tip: do not hang your heavy bag directly beneath your wife's china hutch upstairs. The reverberations from hammering the bag can ripple throughout the house's substructure and rattle the dishes and nerves of everyone inside.

EXERCISE FOR THE BODY AND THE MIND

I've got a yoga mat and a DVD on tai chi—one of these days I may actually use them. Meditative exercises are really very good ways to work out by strengthening the mind and body at the same time. Years ago, I was a fairly accomplished practitioner of yoga, and taking up yoga again is part of my master plan.

COMPUTERS

You can't exactly surf the Internet or build electronic spreadsheets without a computer, but you still can lose weight and reclaim your health without one. If you do have a computer, use it to become a better, stronger, and healthier person, not as something to sit in front of all day long.

Oh yes, there's one other computer I need to mention. I'm talking about the one between your ears: your brain. That lump of grey matter that fills up what would otherwise be an empty space for rent is without a doubt the most important tool in your arsenal. Like your muscles, it too can go flabby and limp, so you've got to keep it toned. Repeat after me: "Read, think and learn; read, think and learn." Do that often enough and your brain will be as taut and brawny as the rest of your body.

Exercise does a body good, but only if that body is properly fueled. After years of eating all the foods that were wrong for me, I had to learn through trial and error what worked best. One of the most important things I learned is that food is so much more than just fuel for the body. The food we eat is part of our cultural identity, a link to our past and a path to our future. The quality of our food plays a significant role in the quality of our lives. Is it any wonder, then, that at one time in our collective history, food was sacred?

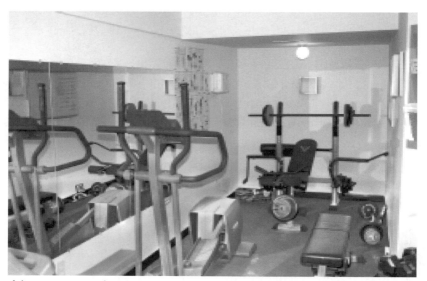

A home gym can be set up in any room. The goal is to create a space that is dedicated to exercise—just as a kitchen is dedicated to cooking or a home theater is dedicated to entertainment.

Part Four
It's All About the Food

Chapter Eleven

When Food Was Sacred
Remembering when food was an important part of our lives

In 1979 when I was in college, I borrowed three hundred dollars and bought my first car, a pea green, four-door 1970 Datsun. The previous owners accessorized the paint job with a collection of dents that covered the car like chicken pox. The rear end had been smashed in an accident, making the trunk nearly unusable. The tires were bald, the stick shift flopped about dangerously and sometimes popped out of gear of its own accord, engine fumes leaked into the passenger compartment, and occasionally the car suffered a seizure and shook so violently that it was impossible to steer.

Like most college students, I was a pauper and could not afford many of life's little extras. I had to save money wherever I could and one of the ways I saved was on gas. I generally gassed up at stations where the prices were the lowest and the quality poor. I'm not saying the proprietors of these fine establishments watered down their gas, but judging by all the knocking, stalling and backfiring that ensued, I came to the conclusion that my gas tank contained more than just fossil fuel.

To make ends meet, I worked a part-time job at a large print shop. One day, at the end of my shift, my car ran out of gas in the parking lot. One of the forklift drivers came over and offered to give me enough gas to get home. He disappeared around a corner and came back a few moments later with a large fuel can. This was the same gas we used in the company trucks and it was the good stuff, premium quality, the fuel equivalent of a fine wine.

The car started up immediately. That didn't happen very often. On my way home, the car ran more smoothly than it ever had before. The engine fairly purred. As I sat at a stoplight and marveled at the low throaty growl of what sounded like a high performance engine, I closed my eyes and imagined I was driving a Mercedes or some other luxury dream machine. My ancient, ailing Datsun, a true automotive embarrassment, was now transformed into a prowling cat of a car, quick off the line and tight in the turns. As there was only enough fuel to get me to a gas station near my home, those dreams vanished quickly. Once I topped off the tank with the cheap anemic gas I normally purchased, the ghost of my old car returned with the familiar knocking, back-firing and inconvenient stalls.

Now consider the human body. We need food the way our cars need fuel. When we put poor-quality fuel in our cars, we see that decision reflected in poor performance, breakdowns and costly repair bills. The same is true of our bodies. Poor-quality food yields similarly poor physical and mental performance. The difference is that in us this inferior performance manifests as aches and pains, lethargy, mental fog, obesity and a variety of illnesses. People who care about their cars don't fill them up with the lowest quality gasoline. They understand that doing so, over time, can have a ruinous effect on the engine. The same is true for our bodies.

If you want to increase your personal mileage in life and take on the tight turns the world sometimes throws at you, if you want to barrel down the straightway, if you want to look back on your life and say with conviction that yours was a race well run, you had better start filling up on the right fuel right now.

FOOD AS SOCIAL RITUAL

When I was growing up, the purchase, preparation and consumption of food was an important part of our lives. In our home, the value of self-reliance meant that it was just as important for the boys to know how to cook as the girls. Our Thanksgiving meals were elaborate affairs requiring days of preparation. Even on ordinary days, food was not taken lightly. Food was sacred then, and the preparation of a meal was considered tangible evidence of love for fellow family members. The food we ate was woven into the fabric of our social behavior. It gave meaning to the notable events of our lives and was a cornerstone of our cultural heritage.

When illness struck, our mothers were more likely to head for the kitchen than to the doctor or pharmacy. Reliance on aspirin and bottled cold remedies was rare in those days. The front line of our defense against ill health came in the form of citrus teas of boiled grapefruit and black pepper, or—the nuclear weapon of home healing—chicken soup or jellied bone broth simmered for hours over a slow flame. Our mothers were live-in physicians and their medicine cabinet was the kitchen cupboard. A teaspoon of cod liver oil was a regular prevention tactic.

When I was about five years old, I came down with the mumps, an illness characterized by painful swelling of the salivary glands. My mother prepared a heated poultice which was wrapped beneath my chin and knotted atop my head. The unmistakable smell of sardines gave me a clue to what it contained, but to this day I do not know all the ingredients. The important point is that with this remedy and a diet of revitalizing soup, I was soon my old self again. This was in 1965, two years before the introduction of the mumps vaccine.

When Mary was a child, she and a number of her siblings came down with whooping cough. They were promptly quarantined from the rest of the family and put on a rigorous regimen of soup. There was little else they could eat, their throats were so sore. As their health returned, their strength was further boosted with a delicious remedy of fat and protein in the form of scrambled eggs.

During the 1960s the whole country was in a state of transition where food was concerned, but our family still maintained a sense of harmony with the natural world. We ate produce in season and harbored little expectation for ripe tomatoes in the dead of winter. The Southwest has a long growing season, but we still had to wait until the oranges and sweet pink grapefruits were ripe. The culture of convenience and instant gratification had not fully taken over. We accepted a slower pace of life where food was concerned, even if we did not understand its importance.

The milestones in our lives had their own special traditions and their own foods. In our community, elaborate wedding receptions were rare. After the cake had been cut, the bouquet tossed, and the happy couple had motored off to parts unknown, the wedding was over.

Funerals were another matter altogether. After a funeral, it was customary to bring a dish—something cooked in your own kitchen—and gather at the home of the bereaved. There the tears of the morning's sorrowful events were replaced by warm embraces and sincere expressions of sympathy in one corner of the house—and boisterous laughter in another. Food was at the center of these events. People usually brought their favorite dishes and though the food was ostensibly intended for the bereaved, there was always more than enough to feed a houseful of sympathetic family and friends. Food after a funeral was a salve, a tangible sign that warmth and comfort could still be found in a world gone cold with the loss of a loved one.

It would have been unthinkable to bring a bucket of heat-n-eat frozen chicken to a funeral reception. In our home, the same was true for birthday cakes. Our cakes were baked from scratch. I was always overcome with a sense of anticipation when I watched my mother bake a cake. There was the flour, the eggs and the folding of the batter, followed by expectancy as we waited for the layers to bake. There was always the inevitable jockeying to see who got first dibs on licking the sweet batter from the beaters. Then the entire house filled up with the sweet scent of freshly baked cake. First one, then two, and finally three flat disks of cake were stacked on a plate. Sometimes, the layers came out of the oven uneven, but my mother, an accomplished pastry engineer, knew how to shore up an uneven cake with strategically placed toothpicks that became the focus of seek-and-find games when it was time to cut the cake.

The best part of baking a cake was decorating it. Real butter and sugar with chocolate or coconut were mixed together to create a blissfully delicious icing. If I didn't nag my mother too incessantly, I got to help ice the cake and even finish off the remnants in the bowl. To the layer of icing she would add decorative walnuts or chopped coconut. These cakes were culinary masterpieces compared to the manufactured, oversized, store-bought cakes available today. Decorated with icing made from partially hydrogenated vegetable oil mixed with sugar and colored with dyes, they may be appealing to the eye, but these cakes are devoid of character, of any sense of the unique.

More important than the taste was what my mother's cakes represented. Those homemade birthday cakes were a tangible expression of her love for me. The store-bought slabs that pass for cake today are a symbol of so many modern parent-child relationships—superficial style and little substance.

Many children today have never seen their mothers bake a cake or their parents actually cook real food for them. They come home to packaged noodles they prepare themselves in the microwave, or eat dry out of the bag. That personal connection with a parent made possible through food does not exist in their lives. This makes for a sad commentary on the state of relationships; for what does it mean when one person says to another, in deeds if not in words, "You are not important enough for me to cook you a meal"? When the sustenance of our bodies is left to strangers, where then can we look when seeking to sustain our hearts and our minds?

EVERYDAY FOOD, EVERYDAY PEOPLE

Not that many years ago, then, food played an important part in our social traditions. From the youngest children to the weathered grandmothers, the cultural role of food in our lives was as vital to our existence as our faith. The following is a short list of how food was intertwined with the social customs of my youth.

- Young children playing house would often pretend to cook food because they understood at an early age that cooking and eating home-prepared foods were components of the glue that holds families together.
- Preparing a dish, or perhaps dinner, for the first time was a rite of passage.
- While a young man asking a young lady out to dinner was clear evidence of a romantic interest, if she cooked for him, that was an order of magnitude more serious.
- Birthday cakes were baked from scratch because no one could bake as well as mom.
- Homemade, hand-cranked ice cream was a rare treat that was always regarded as superior to store-bought ice cream.
- It was considered a sin to waste food.
- Home-cooked meals were considered superior to all others.
- Women and men bragged about their cooking ability.
- Cooking was considered a necessary skill.

We may have lacked many things in those days, but we ate good food, and, like my old Datsun running on good gas, we were healthier for it. Without a full-time working automobile, money for cabs or even buses, we walked most places. But the food we ate was satisfying and provided the nutrients needed to fuel a day's worth of tasks. Overweight people were rare in those days. We saw obese people in the freak shows at the county fair. There, for the price of a bag of popcorn, one could gawk at the fat lady or the fat man and marvel at the expansive capacity of the human body. Now all one needs to do is go to the mall or look in the mirror. This is progress?

Food used to be simple, but not anymore. The burden of trying to decide what we should eat has turned meal planning into a science project. A quick look at a typical list of ingredients helps explain why. Over the course of two years, I had to relearn a few of the simple things about food, and about what happens to us when we eat.

Chapter Twelve

Just the Facts about Food

A few simple things about food that made
all the difference for my family

There is actually nothing simple about food anymore. The typical grocery store has thousands of items for sale. Most of this food comes packaged in pretty containers festooned with appealing images and text. These foods often contain a worrisome list of preservatives and additives designed to make the food appear fresh. Some of the chief ingredients include sugar, grain, soy, vegetable oils and monosodium glutamate. Let's take a closer look at some typical foods and ingredients.

SUGAR

It has been said that money makes the world go round, but I'm convinced it's sugar that keeps us spinning through the cosmos. Sugar, and sugar substitutes, are the drug of choice today for both children and adults. When I was young, we had desserts made with sugar as a special treat. Not many generations before that, refined sugar was unknown.

Few who experience the taste of sugar for the first time can resist it—and that is the problem. Even in moderate amounts, sugar in all its forms can wreak holy havoc on the human system. When we think of sugar, we often think of plain old white table sugar, but practically speaking, we get sugar in a variety of forms. There's cane sugar, crystalline fructose, high fructose corn syrup (HFCS), corn syrup, honey, tree sap (maple syrup), the natural sugars found in fruits and vegetables, and lactose, the naturally occurring sugar found in milk. White flour and white rice are also a source of readily available sugar in the form of glucose.

When you eat sugar it is quickly broken down and absorbed, arriving in your bloodstream as glucose, which is then transported to your muscles for energy. If you happen to be exercising, this energy is used, but if you're sitting on the couch giving your thumb a workout on the TV remote, any glucose that exceeds the carrying capacity of the liver and muscles gets stored in your adipose tissue—in other words, you get fatter. This whole process requires many vitamins and minerals, but refined sugar provides none of these, so the body has to use nutrients that it has stored. Eating refined sugars is like going to the bank every day to withdraw money without ever making a deposit. Soon your body—like your bank account—becomes depleted.

Another problem with refined sugars is that they are metabolized very quickly, shooting straight to your bloodstream. Your blood sugar goes up, triggering an energy burst and even a drug-like high. This blood glucose spike triggers an insulin response—insulin gets sugar out of the bloodstream by moving it into the cells—so your body can bring the level of glucose back to normal. Then, as blood glucose levels drop, you get the inevitable "low" in the form of lethargy and a lack of energy. That's when you feel hungry and the cravings begin. You wind up overeating because a diet unbalanced toward simple sugars leaves you hungry more often. If you're not running marathons, all of this excess glucose ultimately gets converted to stored energy as fat. The result is that you gain lots and lots of weight.

If this process goes on too long, your body can become less sensitive to insulin, a condition called insulin resistance. If your body continues under siege in this manner, you risk developing type 2 diabetes, a condition in which the body becomes very insensitive to insulin. This means that your blood will be awash in sugar, but your cells will be starving. . . no wonder so many people don't feel like exercising!

Under these conditions, even sources of sugar normally regarded as healthy—like whole grains and fruits—may supply more glucose than the body can efficiently handle. Type 2 diabetics tend to gain lots of weight, especially around the middle. They may even develop Type 1 diabetes. Type 1 diabetics lose the ability to produce insulin altogether. When this happens, rapid weight loss typically follows, because without insulin, the body becomes very inefficient at storing fat. Type 1 diabetics must rely on insulin injections to make up for the insulin their bodies can no longer produce.

THE BODY FACTORY

Simple sugars provide energy, but they have no nutritive value. If you think of your digestive system as a factory and the various components as machines, running those machines always racks up associated costs. In a real factory, those costs would constitute the operating overhead that includes electricity, personnel, machine maintenance, etc. Your digestive machinery, as well as all of your interdependent biological systems, have an operating overhead as well. Everything from the production of saliva, enzymes and stomach acid to the digestive musculature that moves food along the system exerts a cost in terms of energy and the expenditure of nutrients.

A manager of a real factory would never go to work on Sundays and turn on the lights and all the machines when nothing was being produced. Without products, there can be no sales and no revenue. The costs of running the factory without producing any products would eat into the company's overall profits and lead to bankruptcy. Likewise, a diet high in simple sugars that provides few nutrients brings in little return on the investment of running your body's interdependent systems. Ultimately, you may find yourself filing for bankruptcy in the form of obesity, diabetes and heart disease.

GOING AGAINST THE GRAIN

Refined grains used in donuts, pastries and bread behave much the same as sugar. This means that eating a slice of white bread is metabolically equivalent to eating sugar. White flour is what is left over after whole grains have been stripped of their vitamins, minerals and fiber. Without these nutrients, refined grains are more easily and quickly digested. The net effect is the same as eating sugar, namely a quick rush of sugar into the bloodstream.

I discovered that my cravings for sweet foods remained high as long as my consumption of refined grains remained high. When I scaled back on both sugar and grains, I saw the cravings subside. I have since eliminated added sugars from my diet. The sugar I do consume comes in the form of fructose, found in fruits and some vegetables, lactose, found in dairy products, and the rare treat sweetened with raw honey or maple syrup, two sweeteners that still contain all their vitamins and minerals.

What about whole grains? I eat very little grain, but when I do, it's whole grain. However, I discovered that while whole grains are clearly better for me than refined grains, they still exerted a dampening effect on my physical and emotional well being. Overconsumption leaves me feeling lethargic, so I don't eat even whole grains very often. After nearly two years of eating small amounts of whole grain foods, I find that I no longer crave either sugar or grains.

SOY

I was once an ardent admirer and consumer of soy foods. I believed in the much-hyped message about the healthful benefits of soy. I ate flavorless tofu straight out of the package. I consumed soy protein shakes, soy meat and a host of other synthetic foods made from this "miraculous" substance, credited with curing everything from cancer to baldness.

Soy is a potent source of isoflavones, compounds that mimic the effects of estrogen, a female hormone. While the industry claims these isoflavones are beneficial, studies have actually linked them to thyroid problems—and a consequence of low thyroid function is weight gain and persistent fatigue. Even worse, a university study showed that men who were subjected to megadoses of soy experienced breast enlargement, nipple discharge and a reduction in testosterone production. Yet the newspapers touted this study as proof that men should eat more soy!

Chapter Twelve: Just the Facts about Food

Soy has been marketed as a health food for years, but this has more to do with the fact that the soy industry spends millions promoting soy products than any inherent health value. A cursory look at the research reveals a troubling list of health problems from this so-called miracle food. I recommend *The Whole Soy Story: The Dark Side of America's Favorite Health Food*, by Kaayla T. Daniel, PhD, a book that will open your eyes to the downside of soy.

In Asia, soy serves as a flavoring agent and a condiment; in the U.S., soy first entered the food supply as cheap animal feed. But the industry has cleverly marketed cheap imitation foods based on soy as high-end health foods. There's irony here in that really high-end foods and ingredients—like saffron, truffles, fois gras and expensive wines—rarely show up on the average American table.

One of the claims made for soy is that it is "natural." This is true only insofar as everything on planet Earth derived from raw materials is natural. What's unnatural is the frightening collection of synthetic foods based on soy. Soy "milk," soy "meat," soy "cheese"—the list of fake foods grows every day. What's worse is that these faux foods come bundled with troubling amounts of sugar, MSG, refined grains, processed vegetable oils, additives and preservatives.

Never in the history of the human race have people consumed as much soy as we do today. In many grocery stores, half the space in the dairy case is taken up by soy products. Babies are given soy milk; school lunch programs now include foods "enhanced" with soy; and most processed foods contain soy as an ingredient. Yet no one knows how a dietary change of this magnitude will affect the populace over time. In animals, soy feeding leads to infertility, thyroid problems and liver disease. While traditional fermented soy foods—the kind of foods Asian societies have consumed for centuries—are historically safe when consumed in small amounts, overconsumption of processed soy foods is a potential Pandora's box of unpleasant surprises twenty or thirty years from now—or even sooner

Despite my many years of devotion to soy, I immediately stopped eating it when I learned about the downside. When I exorcised soy from my diet and converted to real food, many of the dietary demons that had haunted me for more than a decade were vanquished.

FATS AND OILS

I do not avoid fat, but I'm careful to eat only the right kind. That means mostly animal fats, the traditional fats that have sustained humans for thousands of years—real butter, lard rendered from healthy, humanely raised pigs, whole dairy products, whole eggs from pastured chickens, the fat on my meat and good, old-fashioned cod liver oil. As for the oils that come from plants, I use coconut oil and a little olive oil. Nutrition professionals will tell you that you should not consume these fats because, with the exception of olive oil, they're bad for your heart. This position defies logic because for thousands of years human consumption of these fats was commonplace and heart disease was practically unknown. What was really bad for my heart was carrying around an extra two hundred pounds that I couldn't get rid of because of a lowfat, processed-food diet that left me undernourished, enervated and depressed.

When I was younger, my mother used to render lard by boiling fatback. When she was in her forties, her doctor told her she would die of heart failure in a year or two, yet she lived a vigorous and full life well into her seventies. She died several days after paying a long-delayed visit to a doctor where she was subjected to a round of supposedly "necessary" inoculations.

For an eye-opening, science-based explanation of why the cholesterol and saturated fat theory of disease doesn't hold up, read *The Cholesterol Myths*, by Dr. Uffe Ravnskov.

A few decades ago, we were advised to switch from healthy animal fats to vegetable oils. We were told that these mostly polyunsaturated oils were healthier for us. Yet highly polyunsaturated vegetable oils are full of what's called free radicals, the real culprit in cancer and heart disease. And when these liquid oils go through a process to make them hardened—called partial hydrogenation—trans fats are formed. Like the free radicals in vegetable oils, trans fats contribute to cancer, heart disease and many other ailments.

There are many good scientific reasons for eating traditional fats. Animal fats provide important nutrients you can't get anywhere else, including one called CLA (conjugated linoleic acid), which occurs in the fat of grass-fed animals. CLA has been shown to help the body lose fat and build muscle. Lard is a great source of vitamin D, and butter and egg yolks from grass-fed animals provide vitamin A. As for coconut oil, the body uses much of the fat in this extraordinary substance for quick energy and never stores it in the fatty tissues. Coconut oil also boosts thyroid function, making it a great fat for weight loss. The good fats in coconut oil are all saturated fats. When the anti-saturated fat hysteria came along, the food industry was forced to switch from lard and coconut oil to partially hydrogenated vegetable oils loaded with trans fats.

I love to cook with coconut oil because it provides an excellent source of energy, adds tons of flavor to food and acts as an appetite suppressant, which helps spur weight loss.

If you want to know more about coconut oil and its healthy role in diet and weight loss, read *Eat Fat, Lose Fat*, by Mary G. Enig, PhD, and Sally Fallon. Another book, *Know Your Fats: The Complete Primer for Understanding the Nutrition of Fats, Oils and Cholesterol*, by Mary Enig, is the most comprehensive, unbiased and accurate book on the science of dietary fat available to the public.

As for olive oil, I consume small amounts of extra virgin olive oil that is packaged in dark bottles (to protect the oil from light). I keep olive oil in a dark cool spot in the pantry, and buy small bottles so that it doesn't sit around for too long. I never cook with olive oil, instead using it as a flavor enhancer on salads and for making homemade mayonnaise.

MONOSODIUM GLUTAMATE

Monosodium glutamate, or MSG, is manufactured free glutamic acid used to enhance the flavor of some of your favorite foods. While the FDA allows the use of MSG in many foods, ongoing research suggests that MSG may react negatively with the human nervous system. Animal studies have indicated that MSG can cause brain damage, yet it still shows up in baby foods disguised as hydrolyzed protein. Some of the symptoms experienced by people sensitive to MSG include headaches, chest pain, nausea, drowsiness and weakness. Most interesting is the fact that giving MSG to growing animals makes them obese! You don't need a degree in food science, chemistry or endocrinology to realize that MSG is an additive to avoid.

A significant problem with manufactured free glutamates is that their presence in food is not always easy to discern, as they may be listed under a number of euphemistic aliases including "hydrolyzed protein," "autolyzed yeast extract," "flavors," "natural flavors," "broth" and "sodium caseinate." There is only one way to eliminate MSG from your diet and your life—eliminate processed foods!

ARTIFICIAL SWEETENERS

Industry acknowledgement of the hazards of excess sugar is reflected in the growing number of artificial sweeteners on the market. However, concern for dietary sugar has mostly been limited to the calories it contains and its effect on weight, not on the nutrients that sugar depletes. Saccharine (Sweet 'N Low), sucralose (Splenda), aspartame (NutraSweet and Equal) and a number of other contenders have vied for the top spot as America's replacement for sugar. Most consumers are unaware of the fact that the safety of these chemicals is questionable. They have been implicated in a host of neurological problems, including migraines, seizures and Parkinson's disease.

People today assume that we need a lot of sweets in our diet. The sensory appeal of sugar and its substitutes is undeniable, but I believe that appeal has been exaggerated by diets overloaded with sweet-tasting foods. I discovered that replacing sugar with sugar substitutes did little to curb my cravings for sweet foods. In some cases, because the substitutes never tasted as good as regular sugar, my cravings for the real thing became even stronger. I realized that my threshold for detecting sweetness was distorted, and that by consuming sugar substitutes I was maintaining an abnormally high level of desire for sweet foods.

Research suggests that sugar substitutes interfere with the body's ability to regulate caloric intake, leading to greater consumption and weight gain. Once I cut out artificial sweeteners altogether and replaced them with small amounts of natural sugar from raw honey and maple syrup, my "satisfaction-threshold" for sweetness dropped dramatically! Sugary drinks became too sweet for my taste, and now when I do consume something sweet—like fruit or ice cream sweetened with honey—a little bit goes a long, long way.

WHY ARE WE SICK?

It should be apparent by now that many of us are eating large quantities of foods that our bodies are not designed to digest. Critics of this view protest that all foods are equal; they suggest that our digestive systems are little more than hollow, biological garbage disposals through which we can flush all manner of junk food without fear of any ill effect save weight gain.

Those who warn about the dangers of an unhealthy diet are scare mongers, say the "experts," while claiming that exercise is a panacea for all our problems. Actually, the true scare mongers are those who deprive us of our right to accurate information on nutrition and the ability to choose what we eat. They do this by undermining the political process through industry-funded influence on our elected officials and government agencies.

Is food the cause of many of our health problems today? Food is not the sole cause, but it is certainly a major contributor. What could have more impact on our health than what we put into our bodies every single day? To suggest otherwise is to separate oneself from reason and common sense.

Chapter Thirteen

What I Eat
A look inside my pantry at the foods that changed my life

The foods that helped my family members regain their health and Mary and I lose over two hundred pounds between us are the same foods that kept my parents and grandparents healthy and slim. You can find these foods today through the local chapters of the Weston A. Price Foundation.

GRASS-FED MEAT

I eat meat from pasture-raised animals, including beef, chicken, pork, lamb and turkey. I get much of my meat from local farmers who care for their animals properly. I've found that grass-fed, pastured beef is far better for me than grain-fed. The chicken and turkey are pastured as well, and the pork comes from a trusted source. And I eat these meats with the fat—all the fat on the beef, lamb and pork, and the skin on the chicken and turkey.

I believe the quality of the meat I eat is very important. When the grocery store is my only option, I buy meat there, but not processed meats like sliced turkey, ham and beef. These meats are often loaded with MSG and sometimes sugar. When I do buy meat from a grocery store, I buy from the butcher. If you can afford it, consider purchasing a half or quarter of pastured beef. You'll need plenty of storage, but the price break you receive for buying in bulk makes it worthwhile to purchase a freezer.

A Life Unburdened

Once when I was child our home was burglarized. We found that the usual items had been taken: a camera, radio and a few other small electronics. What surprised us was the discovery that several packages of steak, from a side of packaged beef we kept in the freezer, were also missing. It seems that even petty thieves understand the importance of nutrient-dense foods.

I also enjoy organ meats, principally liver, and eat it several times a month. Cow's liver is nutrient dense, and when cooked properly, that is to say rare, it is delicious.

SEAFOOD

We eat many types of fish and I try to purchase the whole fish so I can use the heads and carcass for fish stock. I buy wild-caught salmon when I can get it, but will settle for farm-raised in a pinch. I have found sardines to be an excellent seafood source, and take tins with me when I travel.

Shellfish such as crab, lobster, shrimp, mussels and oysters are extremely nutrient dense and deserve a place in a healthy diet. The oysters can be eaten both raw and cooked.

RAW DAIRY

Imprison a milk cow in a confined space, force her to stand on concrete, keep her strung out on hormones and antibiotics, and feed her nothing but grain, soy and bakery refuse. How can you expect her milk to be nourishing? I've touched on this point before, but I want to talk about one of the foods that has been essential in my recovery. Milk from these "factory" cows is pasteurized and homogenized to produce a beverage that is nutritionally inferior, difficult to digest and uniformly bland throughout the year. This triumph of "consistent mediocrity" is regarded as a success by the industrial milk industry.

Pasteurized milk is milk that has been quickly brought to high heat to kill pathogens that may be lurking in the milk. This is a necessary step with commercial milk from factory-farmed cows, which is typically brimming with pathogens. Unfortunately, pasteurization also kills off the beneficial bacteria and enzymes in the milk, making all the nutrients more difficult to absorb and turning it into little more than dead, white water. Actually, most milk today, including "organic" milk, is ultra-pasteurized, that is, brought to a temperature above the boiling point in just a few seconds. More and more people simply can't tolerate commercial milk. I can't. It literally makes me sick.

The alternative is unpasteurized milk from a cow that grazes on green pasture on a family farm. In fact, the healthiest milk (and butter, cream and cheese) comes from cows eating new grass, growing at an accelerated rate in the spring and early fall. Taken in raw form, milk from these cows is full-bodied, much creamier, easy to digest and incredibly delicious. The fast-growing grass is more nutrient-dense and undoubtedly more delicious to the cows. Butter made from this milk is flavorful and has a rich golden color and an aroma you can smell from across the room. By comparison, conventional butter from pasteurized milk has no aroma at all. But the real difference is in the nutrients. Butter from cows eating grass has many more.

Whipped cream and ice cream made with cream from cows eating green grass have superb flavor and texture. Once you partake of this ambrosia, you begin to appreciate the concept of "living off the fat of the land." I also consume delicious raw cheese and yogurt made from raw milk.

Raw milk is actually quite safe as long as the farmer follows reasonable standards of cleanliness, because raw milk contains many components that kill off harmful bacteria. In addition, raw milk directly purchased from a pasture-based farm comes from cows allowed to graze on grass, not kept confined in sheds and not fed growth hormones. Because these cows eat the food they were designed to eat—grass—they are typically disease-free and do not require antibiotics.

Raw milk—Nature's perfect food—may not be an option for everyone because pressure from the dairy industry has made it illegal to sell raw milk in a number of states. However, it is becoming more available, and with a little effort you can probably obtain it. The web site realmilk.com lists local sources in your area including milk available through cow-share and herd-share arrangements. (A cow-share program allows you to become a co-owner of a cow and drink your own milk from that cow.) You can even order raw milk from farmers who will ship it to you frozen.

It is a sad commentary on the state of the nation when citizens who wish to purchase good, clean, healthful and delicious raw milk are prohibited from doing so by an overzealous regulatory system that fears the healthy competition from raw milk sales. Raw milk may not be for everyone, but everyone should have the right to drink it if they want to.

EGGS, WONDERFUL EGGS

Like many people today, I had a mortal fear of eggs. I believed the myth that they were dangerous due to their supposedly unhealthy combination of dietary fat and cholesterol. Since I still liked eggs, I resorted to some of the egg now substitutes available. But I found that if it looks like an egg and cooks like an egg, it doesn't necessarily taste like an egg. I was not impressed by the egg substitutes I tried. I later learned that when egg substitutes are fed to rats, the animals die very quickly.

In time I discovered that blood cholesterol levels are minimally affected by dietary cholesterol, and that the theory of cholesterol as a primary cause of heart disease is unsupported by science. Now I eat eggs often. They really are a perfect food. My preference is for pastured eggs, which are eggs from chickens that spend lots of time on grass, socializing, exercising, developing a pecking order and eating greens and bugs. I've found that the darker the egg yolk, the more flavorful and nutritious the egg. Spring yolks from pastured chickens are deliciously dark—almost orange. Conventional egg yolks are woefully pale in color and taste. Nevertheless, I much prefer conventional eggs to egg substitutes, which I can no longer abide.

I am somewhat skeptical of terms like "free range" and "cage-free," as I've found these eggs to be only marginally better than conventional ones, as far as taste and color are concerned. I have learned that these eggs come from hens that "roam" in large barns—not in cages, but not outdoors either. If you're going to pay premium prices for any eggs, the first choice should be pastured eggs directly from a farmer. My second choice would be "free range," "cage-free," or "omega-3" eggs. How you eat your eggs is up to you. Whether you like them poached, fried in butter or bacon fat, scrambled in omelets or hard-boiled, it's all good eating.

SOUPS AND BROTH

Two of our favorite foods when the weather turns chilly are soups and broths. A hearty chicken or beef soup that simmers in a slow-cooker all day fills the house with a wonderful aroma and soothes both body and soul. We allow broths to cook for 24 hours or more. Once chilled, the broth changes from liquid to a gelatin. It has been our experience that broth made from the typical big-box grocery store chicken will not gel sufficiently, suggesting a thinness of character to match the deficit of nutrients in these factory-farmed jailbirds. Do not be dissuaded, however, from making your own broth from the chickens you normally buy, as homemade broth always trumps the store-bought variety, which often come loaded with MSG. Broth is loaded with nutrients that detoxify and heal, it is delicious, it possesses magical curative properties. It can be heated and consumed as is or used in soups, sauces, gravies, chile and stews.

FRESH PRODUCE

Anyone who has ever bought produce has encountered the attractive piece of fruit that fails the taste test. When I was a child, it was customary for my family to purchase a large box of red delicious apples during the holiday season. We put these apples out on the back porch where the chill evening air kept them crisp and fresh tasting. It was unusual to find a bad apple in those days. Sadly, the opposite is true today, where finding a red delicious apple that lives up to the second half of its name is a challenge.

Fresh vegetables and fruit are a must in any healthy diet. I eat far more vegetables than fruit, as I've found that less is best when it comes to sweet foods. Finding good quality organic produce is easy, as it is available in many stores these days. Organically labeled produce is nice to have, but don't pass up locally grown produce which, even if it isn't labeled as organic, may be just as good or better. Even conventionally grown fruits and vegetables are superior to anything in the snack food aisle, so don't let the lack of an organic label deter you.

One of the problems with produce in general, and conventional produce in particular, is that growers tend to emphasize size and color over taste. The nutritional value of conventional produce is usually a low priority. The nutrients found in produce are derived from the soil in which they grow. Nutrient-poor soil equals nutrient-poor produce. Poor soil management practices favored by some growers have resulted in produce with reduced nutritional value. This diminished quality in the food we eat is the price we pay for getting what we want exactly when we want it, in or out of season.

When you buy produce in season the prices will be lower and the quality higher. Community Supported Agriculture programs (CSAs) and farmers' markets are an economical alternative for this very reason. While you can save money on conventional produce from the grocery store when items are on sale, your savings are limited by the fact that some of that produce may not be of the best quality.

Local farmers' markets are good places to buy produce, but don't assume that because the guy operating the produce stand is wearing jeans and a straw hat you're getting high-quality, locally grown produce. If it's November in North Dakota and you find bananas and strawberries at the farmers' market, you can be sure those fruits were not locally grown. When in doubt, ask. Buying imported produce isn't inherently bad, but fruits and vegetables grown locally and bought in season usually taste better and are more nutritious. One clue to nutritional quality is how long a piece of fruit lasts. Fruit grown in poor soil rots very quickly.

Why limit ourselves to eating in season? After all, many nutrition experts tell us not to deprive ourselves. They are full of praise for our culture of instant gratification, where nothing is off limits. We're told that human progress is measured not by the realization of our symbiotic relationship with the rest of life on this planet, but by whether or not we can get pesticide-soaked, genetically modified strawberries in the dead of winter to put on our lowfat soy cheesecake.

Eating in season helps us to relearn the virtue of patience and the value of respect for the seasonal growing cycle. Eating in season puts our bodies back in synch with the natural world from which we came. And since there's no such thing as a junk food season, eating in season teaches us to recognize what is and isn't food. In a more practical vein, produce consumed in season typically costs less than higher priced off-season produce. In addition, by buying local, you're supporting the local economy and local growers. Of course, you can always grow your own, and it doesn't matter whether you have forty acres or a few square feet on the back patio of a townhouse, you can grow food almost anywhere.

If you're new to growing your own, farmers' markets are a good place for the beginner to get a jump start on the season by purchasing starter plant. Simply transplant them into your garden. Generally speaking, I've found starter plants from the farmers' market to be healthier and more reliable than those found at the garden centers of big-box stores, and more successful than starting my own plants from seeds. Of course you will expend more physical effort tending your garden, but that's a good thing as the exercise will get you into the fresh air and help you lose weight. The exercise and the satisfaction of knowing that you're eating home-grown, fresh, better-than-organic produce makes that effort worthwhile.

Our garden is a raised bed consisting of two rectangular boxes. Raised beds are great for small gardens because the deep soil provides plenty of extra growing space for plant roots. Longer stronger roots yield bigger, healthier plants. We've had two seasons with our garden where we grow tomatoes, cabbage, peppers, zucchini, onions and collard greens.

Salad vegetables can be eaten raw, dressed with a homemade dressing. Vegetables that you cook are the perfect vehicle for butter and cream!

LIVE FOOD, DEAD FOOD

I also eat lacto-fermented foods, like old-fashioned sauerkraut, kimchee, pickles, beet kvas (a fermented drink made from sugar beets) and kefir, which is a fermented milk beverage. Fermented foods are foods prepared traditionally with a fermenting agent like whey, which transforms the sugars into beneficial lactic acid and creates increased levels of natural enzymes and beneficial bacteria. These enzymes and bacteria help digest our food. Since I've been using fermented foods, I find that I no longer get indigestion or suffer from acid reflux.

One of my favorite fermented beverages is homemade ginger ale. The first time you drink it, you realize it's not your father's ginger ale—it's your grandfather's. I make it with peeled and chopped ginger, raw honey, lime juice and whey. It takes several days to brew and is delicious—sparkling, thirst quenching and non-alcoholic.

Another favorite treat is crispy nuts. I usually use almonds or pecans and soak them overnight in salt water. After soaking, I dry them out in a food dehydrator. An oven on a low setting works just as well. The result is a crispy snack that is delicious and easy to eat because soaking helps to break down the enzyme inhibitors that can make nuts difficult to digest. You'll find recipes for lacto-fermented condiments, beverages and crispy nuts in *Nourishing Traditions*, by Sally Fallon and Mary Enig, PhD.

Humans have evolved to coexist with our environment—an environment that includes a host of beneficial bacteria that aid us in a number of ways, including the efficient digestion of our food. Unfortunately, much of the food we eat today has been stripped of its life-giving properties, foods like pasteurized milk or pasteurized pickles—which are essentially a dead products. Without the aid of beneficial enzymes and bacteria, our bodies must work harder to carry out the metabolic operations they are designed to perform. This extra effort, under less-than-ideal circumstances, wears down our bodies, and causes premature aging, fatigue and disease.

Chapter Thirteen: What I Eat

. . . .

HOME COOKING

One of the great tragedies of modern life is the fact that people no longer cook for themselves. Cooking your own food allows you to control what goes into it, and you can customize your meals so that they are healthy and taste the way you want them to. The biggest lie the food industry has fed to the American public is the notion that we are all too busy to cook. When I consider my wife's mother, who had twelve children, and how she managed to cook meals all those years, I can't understand how my wife and I had so much difficulty getting a homemade meal on the table for ourselves and our two children. Fortunately, we have changed. Either my wife, my daughters, or I have cooked nearly every meal we've eaten since our epiphany in 2003. It took some planning initially, but the challenge was never a lack of time so much as it was a matter of priorities.

THE OBESITY EPIDEMIC

Has an increase in the consumption of sugar, grains, and vegetable oils led to an increase in obesity? Yes, it has. Let's look at the state of food today:

- There are vending machines in public schools, in the workplace and even in hospitals, which weren't there a few decades ago.
- Fast food eateries exist on practically every corner now and can even be found in hospitals. In some inner-city neighborhoods, the only food you can buy is fast food because there are no grocery stores.
- People used to take the time to bake cakes for birthdays. Now you can purchase a massive slab of cake, personalized with a special message, for relatively little money, and in no time at all.
- The pricing structure for junk food is such that for a small increase in price, a customer receives a significantly larger amount of food.
- Government subsidies for corn and soy have fueled explosive growth in the manufacture and availability of cheap junk foods.

- Junk food advertising to adults and children has increased dramatically.
- While gas, housing and transportation costs have risen over the years, the price of processed convenience food has remained constant, or has even decreased.
- Portion sizes in restaurants and in packaged, ready-to-eat convenience foods have increased.
- In every bus station, train station and airport, you can easily find low-cost junk and processed foods, while fresh fruit or real cheese is rarely available.
- Despite the fact that real food amounts to little more than produce, meat, fish, good fats and dairy products, there are thousands of new convenience foods available that didn't even exist fifty years ago.
- Breakfast has degenerated from meat and eggs to sugared cereals to donuts to candy bars. Each successive generation in the devolution of breakfast is higher in calories and lower in nutrients.
- Most of the foods in the grocery store have sugar, grain (corn, wheat and rice) and processed fats and oils as key ingredients.
- It is possible today to buy fifty pieces of fried chicken for as little as twenty-five dollars at some stores. Most of the calories in that chicken come from the breading and the frying oil.

It is an exercise in self-delusion to claim that the modern diet has not caused our current health crisis. The rate of obesity did not double over the last thirty years because people were eating too much fruit, vegetables, meat and whole grains. It doubled because of the reasons stated above, along with a lack of exercise.

In the first half of 2003, my diet and that of my family was as bad as it could be. We were sick and were growing sicker each day. Something had to change. They say that when you reach the end of your rope, you only have two options: let go or start climbing. We decided to climb.

Chapter Fourteen

The Total Food Index
A common sense tool to help you decide what you should eat

I've recently realized that there is a category of food designed to be consumed unconsciously. Put simply, this class of foods is eaten without thinking, like when you're navigating rush hour traffic, juggling a phone in one hand and a quarter-pound burger and fries in the other. Many people will consume this pre-dinner "meal" in their car without thinking, and then sit down to dinner once they get home. That's the magic of these foods. You eat more because you're not fully conscious of what and when you're eating. Our homes, cars and offices are often full of snack foods that we thoughtlessly consume throughout the day. The last thing junk food companies want is for you actually to start thinking about what you eat. Tracking your food neutralizes one of their most potent weapons against you.

But isn't tracking what you eat a lot of work? Not really. Food tracking is not for everyone, but it is useful for some people. Look at it this way: you can continue to be a snack zombie for the food industry or you can wrest back control of your life with this simple, powerful tool. I never would have had any success without this technique. Its power lies in the fact that it puts a halt to unconscious eating. Once you start writing down what you eat before you eat, you will never again put a morsel of food in your mouth without thinking about it first. This technique is a real eye-opener. You may find that you're putting away far more calories or doing much more snacking than you realized. This brief moment of awareness can make all the difference between inhaling a bag of chips and developing the motivation and the good sense not to.

For those people who say, "but I really don't eat that much," consider this: I was socking away well over five thousand calories a day at one point but never realized it. I actually believed I was a light eater most days. The simple fact is that it's awfully hard to pack on one hundred extra pounds without eating a whole lot of high-calorie food.

It is true that as your body becomes more efficient at fat storage, the less you need to eat to gain weight. Still, tracking gives you a baseline of where you're starting from and helps you to see patterns between what and when you eat, your mood and other behavioral signals that can clue you in to some of the underlying emotional, physical and situational reasons behind your eating behavior. If you're eating a good balance of nutritious whole foods, don't be obsessed with macronutrients. The goal is to determine how you ate before you changed to a whole foods diet, and how afterwards. The good news is that food tracking is not something you'll have to do for the rest of your life. For many people, it may simply be a good place to start.

WHICH FOODS SHOULD YOU EAT?

Once you get past the propaganda of "no bad foods," you have to decide which foods you should eat, which foods you should cut back on and which foods to remove from your diet. I devised an effective method for determining which foods I should eat. It may be useful for you as well. I look at food as having four primary properties, which together I define as the Total Food Index or TFI. The TFI rating of any food is a combination of a Nutrition Index, an Accessibility Index, an Addiction Index and a Feedback Index.

The Nutrition Index is the first and most important factor to be considered. Your goal should be to eat the most nutritious foods, most of the time. This index works on a ten-point scale, with -5 indicating the lowest level of nutrition, and +5 the highest. The core question is, how nutritious is a particular food? Foods in the minus range are foods that represent poor nutritional choices, namely processed junk foods. A food rated 'o' would be one that has a neutral or average nutritional value, like homemade cookies containing whole oats and honey. They are nutritionally better than commercial cookies, but they're still not something you'd want to eat every day. On my scale, soda rates very low, with an index of −5, but raw milk, with its energizing enzymes and healthful fat, a +5. I also take into consideration the amount of preservatives and additives in a food. The more of these "extras" a food contains, the lower the nutritional score.

I rate luncheon meat, full of additives, a -2 or -3. Fresh meat gets a +2 or +3 and liver, which is a very nutrient-dense food, gets a +5. Another +5 is cod liver oil. Vegetables are not actually very high on the Nutrition Index, they rate about a +1. However, if you add butter or cream to cooked vegetables, or a homemade dressing containing egg yolks, cream or blue cheese to your salad, the Nutrition Index goes up a point or two.

The Accessibility Index is also a ten-point scale, with -5 indicating the least accessible foods and +5 being the most accessible. The core question is, how accessible is a particular food? In this case, raw milk would rate a −3, as it is not easy to find these days. Soda is everywhere, cheap and readily available, so it would rate a +5. Most processed convenience foods are cheap, easy to find and easy to eat, meaning their accessibility index will usually be high. Another useful example might be a homemade dish like baked salmon. The cost of salmon, plus the fact that you have to cook it yourself, means that you're less likely to eat it everyday. Likewise, if you have baked salmon at a restaurant, the cost and the logistics involved in getting to the restaurant would mean that the accessibility index is lower. Compare the accessibility of salmon to a fried-fish sandwich at the drive-thru. Because fried fish is cheaper, pre-cooked and conveniently located at the fast food joint down the street, the accessibility index will be higher. Not surprisingly, many of the most non-nutritive foods tend to be the most accessible.

The Addiction Index is a ten-point scale with -5 indicating the least addictive foods and +5 the most addictive. The core question is, how difficult or easy is it for me to control my consumption of this food? If you can't be trusted around chocolate, you would give chocolate an addiction rating of +4 or +5. Beef liver from grass-fed animals is a very nutritious food, but for someone who doesn't like liver, the addiction index for liver might be very low (-1 or −2) because they have no difficulty controlling their consumption. Addiction is never a good thing, because it is possible to over-consume healthy foods too, so any food with a high addiction index is something you should manage carefully.

The Feedback Index refers to how the food makes you feel emotionally and physically. Do you get a stomach ache after eating certain foods? Do some foods leave you feeling depressed, while others leave you energized? The feedback index is a ten-point scale with -5 identifying the foods with the least positive feedback and +5 the most positive. I found that keeping a food journal was helpful in determining the feedback index of the foods I ate.

HOW THE TFI WORKS

The primary purpose of the TFI is to help you learn to eat foods that are highly nutritious most of the time. It will help you cut back on foods that are moderately good for you and eliminate those that provide poor nutrition.

Here are two examples of how I used the TFI. Nuts such as almonds are healthy snacks. On the TFI scale for me, they rate high nutritionally (+4), and their accessibility rating is low (-3) because I have to soak them in a brine, then dry them out. The addiction index for almonds is a +2 (down from +5). I used to have great difficulty controlling consumption, so I had to cut back on preparing them. The feedback index was low initially because I found them difficult to digest. Eating them left me feeling bloated. Soaking solved that problem.

Pistachios have a high addiction index (+5) for me. I had to cut them out completely, because I could not stop eating them and the more I ate, the more I wanted. At one time, potato chips were a high-addiction food for me. I'm no longer addicted to them, but because of their low nutrition rating, I don't eat them. The addiction index helps you identify these foods and then regulate their consumption or get them out of your life.

One final example is homemade ice cream. I love it, but the sugar makes the nutritional index for ice cream a -1 for me. Fortunately, because it is made from real ingredients, it is a very satisfying dish, so a little goes a long way, which means the addiction index is very low (-4). With a low accessibility index due to the ingredients required, there's no danger of overeating. I eat about one cup of homemade ice cream per month, and I can enjoy it without worrying about my health.

Why don't I just produce a master chart that shows the TFI ratings for common foods? Wouldn't that be easier? No, because the TFI index ratings will differ from person to person. And while the nutritional indices will remain constant, the accessibility, addiction, and feedback indices may differ greatly. In addition, the TFI rating for a particular food may change over time. You may discover, as I did, that foods that were once difficult to manage are no longer a problem. The most important goal is for you to learn to make these assessments yourself. Investigate the nutritional value of the food you eat. Assess the accessibility and addictive potential of that food. Assess the feedback of the foods. How do they affect you mentally, physically and emotionally? Learn to make the decisions that are right for you. This is the definition of nutritional empowerment.

WHAT'S NEXT?

Eating good food, losing weight and exercising is great, but doing these things just for the sake of doing them seems an empty, unfulfilling activity. I began to see that the business of life is to live, and to live well. In some ways, I still carried the emotional burden of my former life. I needed to be reborn. I needed a challenge, a goal, something to shoot for, but what? I was about to come face to face with the answer to that question—an answer that lay two thousand miles away, spanned fifteen miles and was more than four thousand feet deep. It was time to revisit an old adversary—and friend.

Part Five
Rebirth

Chapter Fifteen

A Day in the Life of a Fit Man

Twelve miles, three thousand feet,
and the challenge of the Grand Canyon

Arizona's Grand Canyon is one of those rare places that is both unremarkable and unforgettable. In 1540, in an area somewhere near the northeastern border of what is now Arizona, the Spanish explorer Francisco Vasquez de Coronado dispatched a group of twelve men to follow up on the claims of their Hopi guides about the existence of a great canyon to the west.

When they reached the Canyon twenty days later, they became the first Europeans to cast their eyes across the great ocean of space. The Spaniards distrusted their eyes regarding the actual size of the Canyon, and so in the manner typical of reckless tourists, they put forth a plan to trek down to the thin sliver of blue that was the Colorado River, which the explorers took to be no more than six feet wide. Hours later, they returned, exhausted, having only made it one third the way toward their goal before realizing the magnitude of their error in judgment. They had discovered what generations of future tourists would come to know: that the canyon exceeds the limits of human comprehension. This is what makes it so unforgettable.

Ever since then, generations of amateur and professional explorers still come, cameras in hand, to document the experience. Unlike the men of Coronado's time, these new explorers return home with color photographs and digital videos to back up their story. It is these innumerable pictures, framed within five-by-seven borders of white or on wall calendars with postcard-perfect images, that become "The Canyon" in the minds of many. Our familiarity with these images is so deeply imbedded in our common memory that upon seeing the canyon for the first time, usually from the popular vantage point of the south rim, the effect can be like looking at just another picture—larger, yes, but completely unremarkable.

When something as grand as the Grand Canyon becomes as commonplace as a postcard, the only thing left to do is venture beyond the rim. To descend into the embrace of these narrow sepia walls is to "see" the canyon with much more than just your eyes. To feel the quickening pace of your own heart, as mind and muscle rally against the inexorable forces of inertia and gravity on the long hike up, is to experience at a gut level what wind, water and time can accomplish.

The first time Mary and I ventured beyond the rim was on a clear morning in September 1986. We had been married less than three months when we decided to make the trip. I was twenty-six years old at the time, and weighed somewhere in the neighborhood of two hundred pounds. As a former weight lifter, I was strong and packed quite a bit of muscle. Mary was twenty-eight and lithe, with an astounding grace, the result of hours of yoga. We were both avid hikers, having spent many a weekend exploring trails from Arizona's arid deserts in the south to the cold mountains in the north.

In those days, we favored a lowfat diet, along with plenty of exercise that included jogging, moderate weight training for me, and yoga for Mary. We were not very particular about where our food came from, and because we kept different schedules and were years away from being parents, we used a lot of processed foods.

It had not escaped my notice that despite my busy schedule and active life, I had steadily gained weight since college. A small "bicycle tire" of fat encircled my waist, and my pants size had increased. I didn't quite know what to make of these changes, as I was clearly not trying to gain weight. Like Boxer, the doomed horse in George Orwell's *Animal Farm*, I believed the solution to my small but growing weight problem was to work harder. I was therefore increasingly determined to avoid fat in my diet and to exercise more.

Another perplexing feature of my health was that despite all the exercise—even in college, when I was running four to twelve miles most days—I noticed that rather than feeling better, the exercise left me in pain. Even though I was trim and solidly muscled at six feet and two hundred pounds, my legs ached miserably after a long run. I took this to be normal, because I had always experienced minor aches and pains after a hard workout. Along with the fatigue, I would often end a long run with a violent coughing spell. I didn't know it then, but I had asthma and it would only worsen over the years. In a feat of irrational logic, I came to accept the aches and pains, respiratory problems and fatigue as the price of being healthy!

The Grand Canyon stretches across the northern end of Arizona for two hundred seventy-seven miles, averaging four thousand feet deep with a six- thousand-foot drop at its greatest depth. The widest point in the canyon spans fifteen miles. The Bright Angel Trail was built by the Havasupai Indians and served as their highway between the canyon rim and Indian Gardens below. The trail is rated as strenuous or difficult by most, and runs twelve miles round trip along the section we planned to hike, from its starting point on the rim out to Plateau Point, six miles away. This section of the trail has an elevation change of more than three thousand feet, with sometimes dramatically changing temperatures between those extremes.

In 1986, we took the Bright Angel Trail down from the south rim, along a series of switchbacks that hugged the sheer walls of the canyon, out to our destination, a dramatic overlook called Plateau Point, which put us about fifteen hundred feet above the Colorado river.

Some experienced long-haul hikers and backpackers consider the Bright Angel Trail to be one of the "easier" trails into the Canyon. "Easy" is a relative term when used in this context. Despite the fact that the trail is heavily used and water is available at several locations, it is a grueling hike. The trip down, while deceptively easy at first, becomes quite the opposite by the time you get to the bottom. Some people refer to the canyon as an inverted mountain, because you climb down first, then climb back up. On the way down you discover that the pitch of the trail and the pull of gravity force you to walk in a crouched, bent-leg manner that ultimately wears out your knees and thigh muscles. By the time we reached the four-and-a-half mile mark at an oasis of cottonwood trees and shaded camp sites called Indian Gardens, our legs were already wobbly from the trip down. We persevered the rest of the distance out to the plateau, where we stopped to rest and enjoy the view. Lunch was a bag of trail mix. It had been cold up on the rim, but down on the plateau, the weather was lovely.

We took some pictures and surveyed the river below, which was brown with sediment. We were in good spirits and spoke about the wonderful dinner we would have upon our triumphant return to the rim. After playing hide and seek with a squirrel, which had apparently staked a claim on this prime piece of real estate, we finally packed our gear and headed back. The first mile and a half on the way back was relatively flat, but once we passed through Indian Gardens and hit the steep trail, we began to experience the Grand Canyon version of hiker's remorse. The hike down had taken a toll on our legs. The four remaining miles up the steep cliffs would test us to the limit. Before long, Mary suffered severe muscle cramps in both legs, her body drained of vital minerals. She could bear no more than ten paces without stopping to rest. I was doing fine for the first mile up, but soon I too began to grow weary.

The last mile was agony for both of us. We must have looked like accident victims to the sympathetic strangers who passed us, many of whom offered words of encouragement. Every step felt as though it might be our last. At about a quarter mile from the top, my left leg cramped up so badly that I could not extend it completely. When we finally reached the rim, instead of celebrating as we planned, we shuffled off in the general direction of our cabin. We were in such a debilitated state that we were quite literally delirious and could not remember where exactly our cabin was.

We stumbled around in the woods for what seemed like forever, until, quite by accident, I found the cabin. When I looked around, I noted that Mary was nowhere to be seen. The selfish instinct to survive had kicked in and I had abandoned her somewhere along the way. Eventually, she found her way back to the cabin on her own.

The sun was still up, so it must have been late afternoon when we arrived back. The odd thing is that neither of us has any recollection of what happened after we made it back. Apparently we showered and changed clothes, but we know this only because when we awoke the next morning, we were in our pajamas. Did we go to dinner as we had planned? Did we talk about our trip and revel in our victory? I don't know and neither does Mary. I ruled out alien abduction as a potential cause of the gaps in our memory and accepted the premise that the hike had essentially transformed us into walking zombies, exhausted beyond consciousness.

The next morning was Sunday, so we decided to attend a sunrise service held on the rim of the canyon. We should have been exultant about our accomplishment and the transforming prospect of attending Sunday services. Instead, we were bundled up in every stitch of clothing we brought with us. While it was cold, and it looked like it might snow, we were a lot colder than everyone else, judging by the curious stares of the other worshippers. Mary could barely walk and shuffled along as if she were recovering from a long and debilitating illness. Her skin pallid, her eyes flat and lifeless, she had the wide-eyed, uncomprehending stare of a prisoner of war who has seen far too much. She mumbled more than spoke and looked as though she might fall over at any moment. I'm certain I didn't look any better.

I don't recall what happened after the service. Did we eat breakfast at one of the hotel restaurants? I can't say. All I do remember is getting into the car and driving past the morning activity on the rim. I have no memory of the five-hour drive home, some parts of which required navigating steep mountain roads, nor do I have any memory of anything else that happened for the remainder of that day.

With the exception of the hike, we blacked out most of the rest of the 1986 trip. We were young and supposedly healthy, but that hike had proved we had a lot to learn about what really constitutes good health. We vowed never to venture "below the rim" again. As the years progressed and our health declined, we became even more certain that we would never hike the Canyon again. Though much of that trip has faded from memory, I treasured what I could remember, because it was all either of us had, and as far as we knew, it was all we would ever have.

RETURN TO THE CANYON

It was the fall of 2004, and I was rolling along on Washington DC's Beltway, Interstate 495, in the always-congested mid-morning rush hour when I had a rather surprising idea. I called Mary and said, "I want to hike the Canyon. It'll be fun and it'll prove that what we've accomplished with our health goes beyond just the window dressing of how we look. It'll prove that we really are stronger and healthier than we once were. Set it up."

Mary remembered enough of our last hike to pause a moment. Then she spoke. "Canyon, the Grand Canyon?" As accustomed to my out-of-left-field announcements as she was, this one startled her. I could hear the incredulity in her voice, but almost immediately, she followed up with a little laugh and an "OK." She knew the difference between my talking just to hear the sound of my own voice and my resolution to follow through on something.

We talked about the trip and the hike later that evening and over the next few weeks. We settled on February 2005 as the date, which left us three months to prepare. There were the logistics to consider, and a half dozen reasons why we couldn't make the trip and shouldn't attempt to hike the canyon. Among them were the weather, my asthma, the five thousand foot change in altitude from our home in Virginia to the Canyon's south rim, jet lag and restaurant food. In the end, all those excuses—and that is exactly what they were—could not stand against the irresistible pull of the Canyon.

My asthma was a serious issue. We would be visiting friends and family in Phoenix three days before our hike. Phoenix is dry and dusty, and contrary to the myth of the desert as a refuge and haven for asthmatics, for me it was a place of torment. During my previous visit to Phoenix, in January 2002, I was only in town for three days, but my asthma degenerated from an intermittent cough to a series of violent attacks. After I returned home, it was several weeks before the symptoms subsided completely. How, I wondered, would I survive two days of breathing the air in Phoenix? Would my asthma symptoms, which had completely disappeared after I changed my diet, return and prevent me from hiking the Canyon?

A second issue was the weather. The prospect of hiking Bright Angel trail in winter was daunting. Just getting to the canyon on northern Arizona's icy roads, which sometimes required tire chains, was a frightening proposition. I was haunted by unpleasant images of our car stuck on a lonely side road in a snow drift, or the thought of slipping on a narrow icy ledge and disappearing over the edge of a cliff in a snow storm.

During the two weeks preceding our trip, the weather forecasts for the canyon played on our emotions, alternating between bright and sunny to cold and snowy. We were in Phoenix when the "final" weather report, two days before the hike, forecast snow for the Monday we had planned for our great adventure. Fortunately, I had passed the asthma test—a good omen.

All the same, I was starting to have second thoughts because of the snow, but Mary reminded me of our reasons for the trip, and so on a brisk Sunday morning, Mary, the girls and I found ourselves heading north on Interstate 17. The weather forecast had not improved. It was worse, in fact, predicting snowfall beginning Sunday night rather than Monday morning. We wanted to be in our hotel before the storm, so except for a stop in Flagstaff to buy crampons (spikes) for our boots, we did not tarry.

Clouds had been building on the northern horizon during the trip and continued to do so all the way to the Canyon. By the time we checked into our hotel, the sky had the unmistakable look of an impending storm.

Snow and ice remained on the ground from an earlier storm. Despite the coming weather and the stinging chill in the air, I couldn't help noticing how different the South Rim is in winter. Gone are the crowds of summer, the jarring chorus of a dozen languages spoken by visitors from all over the world. In winter, one can almost imagine the Canyon as it might have been when Coronado's men first ventured there. Of course, winter also means fewer people on the trail who can help when things don't go as planned.

The El Tovar, the grandest of the South Rim hotels, was closed for renovations. I had hoped to stand before the great fireplace in its lobby and find in its warmth encouragement for the task ahead. Instead, the hotel stood cold and empty against the darkening sky. It reminded me of the dreadful Overlook Hotel in Stephen King's novel, *The Shining*. I couldn't ignore the fact that King's story had unfolded in winter as well.

The view of the hotel was depressing, but the views of the Canyon were spectacular. I looked out over the rim as my eyes tracked the trail all the way out to Plateau Point. Our destination seemed farther than it had been eighteen years earlier.

We found another, less inviting, hotel on the rim. I went to bed that night apprehensive about the coming day.

4:30 A.M.

I awoke early. It was too dark outside to see whether any snow had fallen, but the cold air off the frosted window pane told me it had. The Weather Channel now predicted only snow flurries throughout the day, but that meant it would be cold, with wind chills in the lower twenties. Low temperatures meant that there would be ice on the trail. I did not relish the idea of descending steep and narrow trail on a sheet of ice. Add snow at the upper levels near the rim, and rain beneath the snow line, and we had the recipe for difficulties far surpassing those of our last hike eighteen years earlier, when we were younger and presumably stronger. I began to wonder whether we were getting in over our heads. Soon Mary and the girls were awake and dressed.

Chapter Fifteen: A Day in the Life of a Fit Man

· ·

6:30 A.M.

As the hotel we were staying in had no dining room, we decided to get breakfast at the Bright Angel Lodge. It was still dark, but the crunch beneath our boots provided further evidence of the fresh snow that had fallen overnight. The menu at the restaurant had a so-called "hiker's" breakfast that included cold cereal, fruit and a muffin—a grain-and-sugar recipe for getting stranded at the bottom. Instead, we had eggs cooked in butter with a side of bacon. Mary wanted a breakfast steak, but the only steak on the menu was chicken fried. The waiter acknowledged that the steaks came pre-made and that there was no way to separate the batter from the steak. So much for real cooking.

We rounded off our breakfast with a healthy dose of unrefined coconut oil, which we had brought from home. We also stashed away a second helping in small lidded cups we intended to use once we were on the trail. The coconut oil had hardened to a stiff consistency in the cold climate. I broke off a portion and popped it into my mouth. It had the feel of crunchy candy without any of the redeeming qualities of candy. Though I don't relish the taste of straight coconut oil, I've come to appreciate its appetite-suppressing and energy-boosting properties, and the sense of well-being it creates, so I ate it gladly.

After breakfast, I found a wide-brimmed hat in the gift shop, which was more suitable to wet weather than the knit cap I had brought. As we walked back to our hotel room to get our gear, there was enough light now to see the canyon. To our amazement, it was no longer there. In its place was a sea of clouds that seemed to stretch all the way to the north rim, a sight both beautiful and frightening. Mary and I grew up in the central deserts of Arizona. We were well accustomed to triple digit temperatures that made it hot enough to poach an egg on the hood of your car. But snow, ice and freezing temperatures were not what we were used to. Above us, a second cloud ceiling sent light snow falling.

We were both in a hurry to get going. To stop and think too much about the conditions was to invite doubt and perhaps even failure. We were prepared. We had water, warm clothing, sturdy boots and ski poles and crampons for negotiating the icy trail. Once we had on our gear, we could have been mistaken for experienced winter hikers.

7:30 A.M.

We returned to our room, dressed in our hiking gear and gave final instructions to Stephanie and Raven. They would be staying topside, awaiting our return. Stephanie slumped at the edge of the bed, her posture a study in despondency. I can only imagine what was going through her mind. She had grown up in a sheltered suburban cocoon. It must have seemed to her that we were embarking on an Everest-like expedition where neither success nor life was guaranteed.

The immensity of the canyon and the larger-than-life drama of the storm made Stephanie fearful. I explained that the snow would dissipate once we descended below the snow line, but I could see that for the moment, she longed for the parents she knew when she was younger, the doddering, overweight, TV-watching parents, who could always be found on the sofa, who always made safe, sensible decisions and never took chances. I reminded her that we were the same parents she had always known. We might be thinner and more adventurous, but we knew how to handle ourselves in the outdoors. As I offered these words of comfort, I tried to believe them myself.

We left the room and walked the short distance to the Bright Angel trail head. We put on our crampons and headed down the trail.

8:30 .A.M.

The Bright Angel Trail is made up of a series of short switchback "steps," which in the steepest sections of the trail zigzag along the canyon walls. Opposite the wall, the trail terminates in a cliff that drops off abruptly into the abyss. Switchbacks make the trail much longer, but without them, the trail would be dangerously steep. We cautiously made our way down, using our hiking poles to maintain our balance, and took extra care to dig our crampons into the ice.

To our surprise, we saw tracks in the snow ahead of us, two sets of boot prints. Though out of sight, the other hikers were not far ahead. It was reassuring to see that someone else thought it was a good idea to go for a walk on a morning like this. Maybe we weren't crazy after all.

The going was dicey at first. Once we got over the initial excitement of finally being on the trail, we had to get used to walking with crampons on the steep downhill slope while not getting disoriented by the swirling snow and the stinging cold. While we walked, we talked and took care to follow the tracks ahead of us. Sometimes they hugged the rock-face on the inner side of the trail. At other times, the tracks veered dangerously close to the cliff edge. Visibility was extremely poor in the heavy mist and flying snow. I reminded myself that we could turn back anytime if the conditions worsened. At the same time, I couldn't help thinking that if we could just make it below the snow line, we would be fine.

On the upper trail, the route passes through two narrow, arched tunnels, cut out of the canyon sandstone. During a descent, the first tunnel is a relatively short distance from the start of the trail. The second, slightly larger tunnel is where we caught up with the two hikers ahead of us. They were a tall man in his twenties and a shorter, much older man who could have been in his sixties. They might have been father and son. This is an amazing thing about the Canyon—you meet such a diverse group of people when you venture below the rim. When you see someone on the trail more than twenty years your senior, it's hard to complain about how difficult the hike is. We've encountered many older people on the Arizona trails we've hiked over the years. Our dream has always been to become that "older couple in their sixties," scruffy and muddy, with wide grins, who inspire the "kids" in their twenties and thirties to "just keep on livin'," as Mary's mom likes to say. We bid our fellow hikers good-bye and left them to the shelter of the tunnel.

As we continued along the trail, the snow lightened and the mist began to lift. The temperature became a few degrees warmer, and sleet fell intermittently. We came to icy sections of the trail where we had to place every step carefully to ensure the crampons bit deeply enough to prevent slipping. Eventually, the ice and snow gave way to a frozen sludge, and we could see farther now as the mist lifted and the canyon came slowly into focus, like a black and white photo in a bath of development fluid. The toughest part of the hike was finally over, we thought. We were wrong.

By this time, we were beneath the low-hanging clouds that concealed the canyon from viewers on the rim. The snow had become a light rain which tapped gently on the brim of my hat. The rain was a welcome sign that the ice was behind us. Unfortunately, it also turned the normally dusty trail into a muddy mess. Our crampons were of little use at this stage. We found walking down-slope in mud a tricky maneuver. Every third step or so, our feet would slide in the slippery goo. Step, step, slide, step, step, slide—it went on like this for some time over a series of steep switchbacks known as Jacob's Ladder. Though we had experienced similar terrain in the forested mountains of Hawaii many years earlier, this experience was different. What made it different, and worse, were the mules.

Practically every day of the year, a mule train made up of six or more mules makes its way down the trail behind a guide who invariably looks like an extra from a western movie. Each mule carries one tourist who, depending on his ability to handle heights, is either frightened or delighted. For those people who don't want to walk the trail, the mule train is a great way to see the inner canyon. The rules of the trail dictate that the mules have right of way. When a mule train approaches, hikers are advised to stand quietly by the side of the trail and let them pass.

The mule train we encountered was heading down-trail, as we were. We stood aside and nodded toward each mule and its rider as they passed. The trail, which had been difficult to traverse before, was almost impassible now. The combined weight of the mules and riders had gouged great hoof-shaped holes several inches deep in the mud. The mules also defecated as they walked. The green, steamy piles of mule flop were ground into the mud by the next mule in line, turning the trail into a kind of sticky, stinking, boot-sucking mud pudding. Now, not only did we have to take care not to misstep, slip and go careening off a cliff, but we also had to make certain not to step in any "green mud" as well.

Just as I was beginning to think it might be best to turn around, the rain lessened and the stickiness of the mud subsided. We were on the lower levels of the trail above Indian Gardens, about three quarters of the way on our journey. But now, though much drier, the trail was littered with tennis ball-sized rocks eager to twist my ankle.

10:45 A.M.

We caught up with the mules at Indian Gardens, where the guide had stopped to give the riders a chance to regain some feeling in their rear ends. Indian Gardens is a lovely spot for a break before the trek to the river or Plateau Point. The Gardens get their name from their original inhabitants, the Havasupai Indians, who raised corn and beans here as recently as the early 1900s. A small creek flows through this area making it a tranquil and refreshing sanctuary.

Mary and I decided not to stop here and pressed on instead. The trail to Plateau Point continues on for another mile and a half, where it ends at a dramatic bluff that overlooks the turbulent Colorado River, fifteen hundred feet below. The terrain between the Gardens and the Point is relatively flat and makes for an easy walk. We wanted to get there before the mule train, so we had little time for strolling, and yet the beauty of the Canyon from this vantage point could not be ignored. The ground was carpeted in desert greenery thanks to abundant rain during the previous month. Along the trail, we saw the strangest cactuses, dressed in brilliant purple colors. The canyon walls rose up around us until they seemed to touch the sky. Above us, the cloud ceiling had broken up, revealing a brilliant blue canopy.

11:15 A.M.

I was first to reach Plateau Point, but it turned out I was not alone. I walked to the edge of the rocky ledge to get a better view of the inner canyon and was surprised by the sight of a great black California condor resting on a lower ledge. The bird unfolded its wings to about half mast, a breath-taking sight! Never had I been this close to a condor outside of a zoo. The experience was incredible.

A Life Unburdened

. . . .

Mary and the riders from the mule train soon joined me on the ledge, where we all sat down for lunch. The bad weather had abated, turning what had been an inauspicious morning into a perfect day. We had made it to the halfway point of our journey. Neither snow, sleet nor rain had stayed us from our destination. All that remained was getting back up to the rim. For now, though, it was time to relax and enjoy our meal.

In 1986, at this very same spot, we had consumed a bag of trail mix for lunch. We would not repeat that mistake. We needed a mixture of energy sources in the form of slow-burning carbohydrates, protein and even slower-burning fat to fuel our return trip, so our lunch included homemade beef jerky, a banana, some salted almonds (which we soaked and dehydrated prior to the trip), and a second dose of coconut oil. We washed our meal down with water, then took some pictures and enjoyed the view.

It was difficult for us to grasp the significance of where we were. A year and a half earlier, the only way either of us could have made it to Plateau Point would have been by helicopter. In those days, we both exceeded the two-hundred-pound weight limit set for the mules—in my case by at least two hundred pounds. Standing there with the Colorado River churning below, we celebrated this great accomplishment of rebirth and renewal.

The wind picked up, and we both noticed how cold we had become. The clouds were regrouping above us, and we had several hours of up-canyon hiking ahead of us. It was time to go. We said goodbye to our new friends from the mule train and headed back up the trail.

11:45 A.M.

The walk back to Indian Gardens passed quickly, but about a half mile before reaching the shelter of the Gardens, the storm mounted its second assault. It began with a light rain that suddenly turned into hail. Weather down in the Canyon is generally milder than up above, but here we were being pelted with small stones of ice. Having grown up in Arizona, we knew that hailstorms in the desert were often followed by torrential rains. We quickened our pace. A loud siren went off up ahead in the direction of the Gardens. It was a bit disorienting to hear this mechanical noise amid the sounds of nature.

By this time, the hail had turned into rain, which steadily grew in intensity. As we drew near the Gardens, I looked over my shoulder to see whether I could spot the mule train which had left the plateau shortly after we did. What I saw instead was a wall of water stretching from the heavens to the bottom of the Canyon below. A celestial waterfall roared from the sky, practically obliterating the view behind us. I felt sorry for the mule riders. We had reached the relative safety of a covered information kiosk at the Gardens, but they were still out there. We decided to take a break at the Gardens and see how the storm would play out.

At the time, I didn't know that four-and-a-half miles away, and about three thousand feet above us, the south rim of the Grand Canyon was under siege. Snow was burying everything in sight. A bitter wind whipped the snow into a dancing fury until it seemed as though it was snowing from four different directions at once. Had we foreseen this development, we would never have left our hotel room.

In fact, at that moment, Stephanie was looking out the window and wondering what had become of us. At fourteen, she was the big sister, left in charge while we were away. At the height of the storm, a shrill siren pierced the air and made heads turn in the lobby of the Bright Angel Hotel. Stephanie didn't know what the siren meant, but suspected it wasn't good. As Raven prepared lunch from our store of food, Stephanie pulled the curtains and tried to shut out the cry of the storm.

12:15 P.M.

In the Canyon, the rain finally began to let up. I sought shelter beneath a covered picnic table while Mary made her way back from the rest room. The mule train pulled into Indian Gardens, thoroughly soaked, at about the same time Mary left the rest room. She struck up a conversation with one of the riders. The trail guide had heard a loud boom before the siren sounded, and was checking via walkie-talkie to find out what the trail conditions were. Less than a month earlier, torrential rains had caused a landslide along the upper reaches of the trail, shutting the route down for a time while repairs were made. The prospect of being marooned, even in such a beautiful place as the Canyon, while a storm raged above us on the rim, was more than either of us could bear. Our children were up there! Landslide or not, we weren't going to stick around to find out whether the trail was still intact. We stayed just long enough for Mary to wrap her right knee with medical tape in preparation for the hike up. We checked our gear and set off once again.

12:30 P.M.

As we started out along the rocky trail that lay beyond Indian Gardens, I let Mary take the lead. Her more deliberate pace would ensure that I wouldn't go too fast and burn myself out in the early phase of the return trip. At this point on our 1986 hike, my legs had already gotten shaky from the trip down. Now, although I felt tired, my legs were only slightly fatigued. This was good news. However, the hardest, steepest part of the trail was still ahead of us.

My breathing was a different issue. As we made our way uphill, my breaths came in ragged spurts. I would never make it to the top like this, I thought, so I focused on the early morning wind sprints I ran, in the dark, on the hills back home in Virginia when the temperatures were in the twenties. I reminded myself of "suicide hill," that punishing incline along our favorite bike path, which took me several tries before I could make it to the top without seeming to lose a lung along the way. Pretty soon, my breathing evened out as Indian Gardens fell further behind with each step.

The mule train left Indian Gardens shortly after we did, so it wasn't long before they caught up with us. We stepped aside and found a couple of suitable rocks to sit on, thankful for the opportunity to rest our feet. I was feeling more tired now and knew I was in for a challenge. After the mules passed, we resumed the trail.

It was at this point that I made an amazing discovery. My legs, which had been feeling slightly fatigued earlier, now felt remarkably fresh. What's more, my breathing was calm, and to my surprise, I felt energized. I couldn't believe that a paltry two minutes of rest had reinvigorated me to this degree, but then I remembered the coconut oil. I knew that those medium-chain saturated fats in coconut oil were healthy and provided long-burning energy for difficult workouts, but here I was experiencing the effect in one of nature's most sublime laboratories. I expected my new-found energy to dissipate quickly, as it often did after a short rest on a long hike, but this time it didn't. Like the Energizer bunny, I kept going and going and going. I felt as though I could walk to the canyon rim and keep on going, all the way back home to Virginia if I wanted to. I thought about all the times in the past when I had "carbo-loaded" prior to a run or a workout, thought about the ten-K race I ran years ago and how I ran out of steam halfway through. I had loaded up on carbohydrates for that race while dutifully making sure I avoided as much fat as possible. How could so many people be so wrong about what the human body needs? How, and perhaps more important, why, did we lose our way?

As important as these questions might be, just at the moment Mary and I were faced with a more pressing issue, namely making it back to the rim. We pushed on, stopping now and then for a rest, or whenever the mule train about fifty yards ahead of us stopped so the guide could deliver some bit of Grand Canyon lore. It wasn't long before we encountered the mud again. The rain had stopped, and we discovered that in mud it was easier to walk uphill than downhill. Still, the mud that caked our boots slowed our pace. Each step, in fact, required more energy and put more strain on our weary muscles than if we had been hiking up a dry trail, and the trail was particularly steep in sections.

The inescapable fact about hiking the Canyon is that you have no choice but to climb back out, no matter how tired you might be. Fortunately, Mary and I still had plenty of energy left when we arrived at the part of the trail that was layered with snow. The temperature had warmed the ground sufficiently to turn the ice at the lower level of this section into frozen slush. It's easier to balance oneself when hiking uphill, so we didn't bother putting our crampons back on.

Although the ground was apparently warmer, we felt colder, especially when we stopped to rest, and we were resting more frequently now. Although we had taken care to find the right boots for the hike, we had been less careful in our choice of clothing. We made the error of wearing cotton and cotton-blend clothing beneath our waterproof outer jackets. Inside my jacket, I was sweating like a fountain. Down below in the canyon, that hadn't been much of a problem, but in the cold air above the snow line this choice of clothes was potentially dangerous. We were still at least an hour from the rim—and a warm room and hot shower. By wearing cotton close to our skin, we had violated one of the cardinal rules of winter hiking. Cotton can cause hypothermia. I didn't realize how wet I was, but every time we stopped to rest along the steep icy trail, I grew steadily colder. Mary's hands had become chilled in the frigid air.

At every turn in the trail, I kept hoping we would see some clue that we were close to the top. As we rounded each switchback, I expected to see the arched tunnel we had traversed on the way down. I swore someone had moved it. Although we could see the rim and even people at a distance above us, with each step it seemed to recede. But finally, the tunnel appeared. I almost shouted when I saw it. We were closing in on our goal, but we were also colder and weaker.

Our pace was practically geriatric now. Yet in spite of the long, grueling hours we had just spent, we weren't exhausted. . . but we still had some distance to cover. Those last steps were the most difficult. It is a fact of human experience that the closer one comes to reaching one's goals, the more obstacles get in the way.

The first tunnel appeared before us, and then it was behind us. We could see the buildings on the rim a short distance ahead. We walked the last few switchbacks and emerged, finally, at the top of the trail and the end of our journey.

No marching band, no cheering crowds, were there to welcome us. We hugged for a moment and then kissed. We stared at each other, our faces streaked with rain, our clothes wet and covered with mud. We looked awful, but that didn't stop us from laughing loud and long. We might have looked like two bits on the outside, but at that moment we felt like a million dollars on the inside.

As we walked back to our room we were jubilant. We stopped for a moment along the rim and gazed out at the trail, six miles long and over three thousand feet deep. Even now, it was hard to believe we had actually done it.

We took our time traversing the icy walkways around the Bright Angel Lodge. I was fairly numb by now and simply longed to see my daughters. When we reached our room, I pounded on the door and shouted, "Pizza delivery!" The door opened and Stephanie and Raven exploded from the room and smothered us in excited hugs. It was good to be "home."

Less than two years earlier, we had existed in a crisis state of obesity, high blood pressure, asthma, chronic pain, depression, weakened immune systems and a sense of hopelessness about the direction of our lives. A mere nineteen months later, we were hiking the Grand Canyon. We now knew without a doubt there are no limits to what a willing heart, an active mind, and yes, lots of good food, could accomplish. With this defining challenge behind us, we were finally free to live a life unburdened.

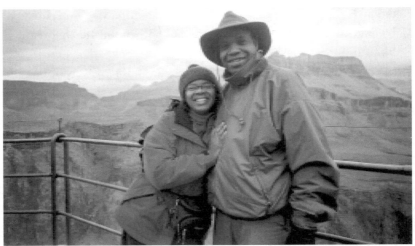

Richard and Mary at Plateau Point in the Grand Canyon, 2005

Chapter Sixteen

Ten Steps to a New Life

Food is key, but recreating your life involves more than just what you eat

Think about the last time you were successful at something. It might have involved achieving an important goal at work or school, or perhaps you landed your dream job or forged a promising new relationship. To achieve this goal, you probably executed some sort of plan. Even if you weren't entirely conscious of a plan, when you review the steps you took to reach your goal, the plan you used begins to emerge.

There's an old saying: "If you fail to plan, you plan to fail." It's true. When you attempt to reach an objective without a clear plan, it is very much like trying to find an address in an unfamiliar city without any directions. While you might stumble upon your destination, it's much more likely that you'll remain lost. Sometimes even with a plan, if it is not the right plan for you, success may prove elusive.

This is how it was with me for years, as I bounced from diet to diet. I followed one plan after another and met with defeat every time. I eventually realized that I needed to take a more proactive role by designing a plan that worked for me, rather than blindly following someone else's plan. This is much easier to do than it sounds. To begin with, you don't have to start from scratch. I didn't. I discovered over the years that even though there was no one perfect weight loss and fitness plan for me, many plans incorporated methods that did work for me. The trick was in identifying those parts of a plan that worked, and knowing which parts to discard.

When I was a vegetarian, I found that a plant-based diet did not work for me, but in the process of making this discovery I learned a valuable lesson about the importance of buying in-season produce. When I tried low-carbohydrate dieting, I realized right away that this approach to nutrition was inappropriate for me as well, but I also discovered a critical need to limit sugar in my diet. In time, I was able to devise an approach to nutrition and exercise that was tailored to my life-style. You can do the same with a little bit of work. You'll discover that just like a tailored suit, a tailored plan for health and fitness will fit you much better, and last longer, than an off-the-rack solution.

Typically, books on diet, weight loss and fitness focus on recipes and exercise routines. These are important components of a successful health improvement plan, but they are not the only components that should be considered. One of the most important things Mary and I discovered on our journey was that improving our health required a multi-disciplinary approach that went far beyond nutrition and exercise. The ten steps listed in an earlier chapter are the same ten steps we used to improve our lives. Here they are again in a slightly different format.

1. Educate yourself.
2. Match the size of the commitment to the size of the problem.
3. Rely on the strength of your tribe.
4. Create harmony in your life.
5. Simplify your life.
6. Eat as though your life depended on it.
7. Make exercise a part of your life.
8. Get plenty of high quality sleep.
9. Find your motivation.
10. Share what you've learned.

Chapter Sixteen: Ten Steps To A New Life

. . . .

STEP 1: EDUCATE YOURSELF

Every successful human endeavor began with a question. Whether it was the discovery of the practical application of fire as a tool for cooking or the landing of a remote explorer on the moon, every accomplishment in the history of mankind began with a single question, fueled by curiosity. This need to know and understand the world around us leads to the acquisition of knowledge, and ultimately, the discovery of truth.

With our busy, modern lives and our insatiable need for instant gratification, we rarely ask questions anymore, relying instead on others to do the work of uncovering the truth. Much like our agricultural ancestors, who forsook the independence of their hunter-gatherer lives for the stability of communal life, we too have come to depend on the "village experts" to ask the questions and provide the sustenance that makes possible our very existence. Our nutritional experts are a diverse collection of doctors, nutritionists, dieticians, food producers and government bureaucrats. Dependence upon these professionals to guide us in making the right decisions about our health is not inherently wrong, but given the sorry state of personal health and fitness in America today, one cannot help but wonder whether the experts are really up to the job.

In times like these, a stiff spine and a frontiersman's penchant for "doing it yourself" are what's needed. That's what this first of the ten steps is about: asking questions and finding your own answers. It's for the professionals to debate the issues, write position papers and attend scholarly conferences in sunny locales to discuss "the obesity problem," but we've got living to do today, and we need practical answers and actionable information now, so let's get on with it.

THE SEARCH FOR KNOWLEDGE

Walk into any bookstore or library and make your way to the diet section. There you'll find hundreds of books on weight management and health. Never let it be said that we are not a health-conscious people! The ever-increasing number of books on the subject of weight loss is a testament to the interest we all have in improving our health and our lives.

And let's not forget the Internet with its gigabytes of dieting information available at the click of a button. You would think, with so much information available, that few people would succumb to a weight problem and the illnesses that follow, yet as a nation we are sicker than we've ever been. Cancer, heart disease and obesity-related illnesses continue to top the charts as our most popular ways to die. The profitability of the pharmaceutical industry, and the rise in weight-related adult disorders like type 2 diabetes in children, is further evidence of the declining state of health in America.

Why, then, with such an abundance of information at our fingertips, have we not been able to stem the tide of obesity and ill health? A line from the book of Hosea in the Old Testament says, "My people perish for lack of knowledge." This quote describes our situation today, for it is a lack of knowledge that condemns many of us to illness and disease. It was a lack of knowledge that was nearly my undoing not long ago.

GETTING PAST "I KNOW"

One of the first things I had to get over was the idea that I already knew everything there was to know about nutrition. Even now, when I talk to people about the importance of learning—really learning—about nutrition and their own bodies, they inevitably reply, "Yes, yes, I know all that, just tell me what to eat."

My reply, when I'm feeling feisty is, "Do you really know?" I'll ask them whether they know the difference between long-chain and short-chain fatty acids and how these fats are metabolized in the body. I'll ask them whether they've ever heard of the Framingham Heart Study and how it has been used both to defend and discredit the cholesterol theory of heart disease, the principal influence behind our present-day dietary policy. I'll ask for their opinion on the merits of grass-fed versus grain-fed beef or what they know about the medicinal value of fermented foods, or even where they stand on the issue of the enteric nervous system as the body's second "brain."

I almost always get blank stares when I ask these questions. I make it clear that my goal is not to belittle, but to point out that the body of knowledge regarding human nutrition does not exist in a vacuum, that it is a complex issue, and that like most complex issues, our understanding of it has been colored by political and economic concerns, which often supersede health concerns.

Only when I admitted I didn't know as much as I thought I did could I start on my quest to discover for myself what kind of dietary regimen would work best for me.

QUESTIONS

So what did I do? First I learned about the foods I was eating. I asked the questions that were relevant for me, then went in search of answers. What was the composition of the foods I ate? How did they affect my body and my mind? How did my enteric nervous system power my gastrointestinal system? How did that system work? What were the different kinds of fats and carbohydrates, and how were they metabolized? What benefits were derived from dietary fat? Was saturated fat really bad for me? Was cholesterol bad or did it provide a useful function in the body? Why was it that after eating a large meal, I'd be hungry again two hours later? Why didn't I have the energy to exercise? When I did exercise, why did I get tired so quickly? Which foods should I eat? Which foods should I cut back on? Which foods should I eliminate from my diet altogether? Why are soy and corn syrup included in so many convenience food products? How has government nutrition policy been affected by politics and economics? What influence do the food and pharmaceutical industries have on what I eat? Why isn't my doctor telling me more? How much of what I know—or think I know—about nutrition, weight loss and processed food is true?

INFORMATION RESOURCES

Information, and lots of it, is the real key to success. You've got to know—I mean really know—why you're following a particular course. Knowledge really is power. If you're simply following some diet guru's advice you will probably fail in your efforts, because blind obedience never lasts long. Real motivation and progress come from knowing about nutrition and fitness and what they mean to you personally, so you absolutely must read, think and learn. And many sources of information are available to us.

The Internet is the place to start. Sure, there's lots of mindless drivel on the Internet, but it's also a gold mine of useful information on health and nutrition. It's hard to imagine that only a decade or so ago, this vast resource did not exist. Whether it's access to medical studies or the rants of real people who have had their stomachs stapled, the Internet is a boundless archive that puts information at your fingertips. See the Resource section for the sites I found most useful.

Don't overlook the public library. Libraries haven't yet gone out of fashion. One disadvantage to the Internet is the absence of a kindly, bespectacled matron to help you find what you need. Libraries are wonderful places to get your hands on medical journals, for example, without having to pay the fee often charged for electronic access. Your local library may also provide free music rentals to give you something to do besides eat while you're driving home in rush hour traffic. You can also pick up exercise video tapes and DVDs at the library or, if like me you've got a thing for salsa (the dance, as well as the condiment), you can check out how-to videos as well. Who says exercise can't be fun? Libraries also host frequent book sales, so there's always an opportunity to pick up something on nutrition, exercise and health at bargain prices.

As for bookstores, many have a bargain table where books have been drastically marked down. Here you can find great deals on health-oriented books. But remember, not everything you read is true or true for you, so be discriminating in your choices. That's where the thinking part comes in. I find it helpful to read opposing viewpoints on a particular subject. That's why reading and gathering information from a variety of resources is so important. If you're only getting one side of the story, you can't make an educated decision.

Magazines and newspapers can also be useful sources of information, but they should be read with a grain of salt. Many of these publications are supported by corporate largesse in the form of advertising or sponsorships. In consequence the editorial position of some newspapers and health magazines has been hopelessly compromised. Examples of corporate influence abound. A popular fitness magazine published an extensive article on the "healthiest" prepared foods. Page after page of highly processed convenience foods were accompanied by glowing recommendations from a panel of nutrition "experts." Amazed, I wondered what kind of nutrition "expert" believes a candy bar is healthy.

A little investigation revealed that all but one of the experts was a dietician. The American Dietetic Association receives funding from a number of food industry interests. Even a casual review of their positions on food and nutrition reveals an organization that espouses a philosophy so close to the food industry's that it is hard to see any difference.

As for television, this is *not* a source of reliable health information. In *The Truth about the Drug Companies*, Marcia Angell, MD reveals one technique for consumer manipulation: the use of celebrities in televised ads, plugging pharmaceuticals while engaging in what appear to be casual conversations. A medium so lacking in ethics that it employs this kind of manipulative marketing should be viewed with skepticism.

Knowledge is just the beginning. Once you begin to understand the basic nuts and bolts of nutrition, exercise and how your own body works, it's time to make a commitment to change. Is a vegetarian diet right for you? What about grass-fed beef, raw milk or fermented vegetables? You'll never know for sure unless you read, think, learn, and explore for yourself.

I believe the secret to improving your health is understanding that no one can do it but you . . . . and you *can* do it! As long as we depend on others (including our doctors) to tell us what to do, we will never make meaningful progress toward our goals.

STEP 2: MATCH THE SIZE OF THE COMMITMENT
TO THE SIZE OF THE PROBLEM

For years, Mary and I purchased one piece of exercise equipment after another. That equipment spent more time as a clothes rack than a workout partner. When we finally made the commitment to build a home gym, we went all out. We invested our money and our time. We integrated the gym into an overall wellness plan that included diet, improving our relationship and finances, and the pursuit of career goals—including my goal of becoming a public speaker.

Making commitments is easy. Sticking to them is work because real progress requires real commitment. This is why the "small steps" philosophy is often unsuccessful—because it's difficult to meet a big challenge with a small solution. I believe you should think big and devise big solutions to solve big problems. Think big when you make your plan, but then execute that plan incrementally—in small steps. But isn't that the same thing as the small steps philosophy? No. Let me give you an example.

Resolving to take the stairs to your office instead of the elevator is a small step which, for many of us, accomplishes nothing. How many times have you taken a small step toward improving your health by buying a diet book, ordering a diet soda or signing up for the free trial period at your local gym? How often did these small steps help you achieve your long-term goals?

The problem is that human beings are task-oriented creatures, motivated by a desire to meet the challenge of long-term achievement. Those achievements can be anything from getting rich to finding love to building a business to helping the poor. Isolated tasks with vaguely defined goals are like orphaned dreams. They disappear once we wake up and have to deal with the real world. So how do we achieve our important goals?

A better approach is to say, "I want to enrich my life, so I'm going to climb Mount Kilimanjaro in Africa next year. To accomplish this goal, I'm going to improve my health and my diet by eating more whole foods, starting today. I'm going to study Tanzania, its culture and people, and

I'm going to get a passport. I'm going to develop a plan that includes meals and exercise with goals for the next twelve months. As the first step in my plan, I'm going to take the stairs to my office every day, starting today." What a powerful commitment that is! As part of a master plan, the "baby steps" approach is a great strategy.

Without a long-term goal, however, a small step becomes an isolated step, unsupported by neither plan nor commitment. But a real goal is a powerful catalyst that lays the foundation for success. Taking the stairs becomes a link in a chain of forward-moving events that speeds you toward your goal.

The major failing of the small-steps approach is that it expects failure, and attempts to counter the potential for failure by reducing risk through the adoption of an approach built upon minimal effort. Goal achievers would call this, "planning to fail." Dream big, plan big, commit big, then execute—in small steps.

STEP 3: RELY ON THE STRENGTH OF YOUR TRIBE

The concept of the tribe—a band of like-minded individuals united in a common goal—is as old as the human race. From the tribe we both derive help and lend support. When we are trying to overcome a health problem such as obesity, we can look to our tribe of friends, family members and medical professionals for help.

I read an article a few years ago about a public figure who underwent a dramatic physical change. He was an extremely "stout" fellow, as they used to say, and I saw in him a kindred spirit who surely understood the burden that I bore daily. Gastric bypass surgery was not the rage then as it is today, so this man decided to lose weight the old-fashioned way, through diet and exercise. As a man of means, he enjoyed the luxuries of a personal trainer and a personal chef. I was happy for him, if not a bit envious. I reasoned that losing weight must surely be a lot easier for someone who has a staff of professionals at his beck and call. I relied on this crutch as an excuse for years afterward, but eventually I had to face up to the fact that my health was *my* problem and *my* responsibility.

Step three of our ten-step plan is all about finding the help you need to reach your goals, even if that help begins and ends with you. The inspiration for this step came in part from a friend who has her own problems with weight. She is a single, middle-aged woman, possessed of a cheerful spirit that brightens any room. Congratulating my wife and me on our success, my friend remarked rather darkly, "It's different when you've got someone to help you." Her comment struck a chord and reminded me of my own similar observation years earlier about the afore-mentioned man of means.

While I am thankful for all the blind luck, blessings and good fortune I've enjoyed, owing to my humble origins I had never thought of myself as privileged. I realized then, perhaps for the first time, that I am, in fact, quite privileged. Financial wealth is a wonderful thing if you can get it, but most would agree that a much greater blessing is the loyalty, if not the love, of another human being. When that love is manifest as a concern for your health and is shown daily in any number of small gestures that assist you on your journey toward wellness, it feels like the Hope Diamond, the Mona Lisa, and all the stars in the heavens belong to you.

We all need a little help from our friends and loved ones, but sometimes that help is not forthcoming. Before we delve into strategies for handling those situations where you find yourself alone in your efforts, let us first look at the best-case scenario, one where you have someone supporting you.

Several popular sayings get to the heart of what it is to be supported by someone: "Two heads are better than one" and "Many hands make light work," are two of them. When my wife and I were doing our initial research on nutrition, we were able to split the work and cover twice as much ground in a short period of time. When it came to exercise, we encouraged each other and, in the first two months when I was still gathering information and grumbling because I hadn't lost the weight I wanted to, she comforted me. I've told her more than once that I don't think I could have made it without her, but at the risk of sounding ungrateful, and maybe even a little arrogant, I know I could have. I believe the same is true for her. Yes, it might have taken each of us a little longer had we gone about this separately, but I believe the solid research we did, as well as the nutritious food we ate, would have ensured our success separately or together.

If you have the support of a friend or family member, coordinate your efforts while eliminating duplication of effort. While one of you researches foods, the other can look into the best exercise routines and equipment. Congratulate each other on your victories, no matter how small, and encourage each other if progress is slow, as it inevitably will be. Most important, be honest with each other. This won't always be easy. When Mary and I first walked the one-mile loop around our neighborhood, our conversations sometimes made us sad and even angry. Without realizing it, we engaged in a year and a half's worth of intensive therapy, walking in circles in the dark and pouring our souls out to each other. Not even the most committed professional counselor will get up at four-thirty in the morning and listen to you go on about yourself the way a good friend or a spouse will. If you have such a person in your life, count yourself among the richest people you know.

Sometimes having more than one person in a household can work against you, especially when one or more members doesn't share your enthusiasm for better nutrition and fitness. When your spouse doesn't share your enthusiasm for healthy eating, improving your diet can be more difficult. In situations like these, compromise is necessary. But even in the best of situations, where you and your spouse agree on most issues of nutrition and exercise, some differences of opinion are bound to remain. People have to learn to negotiate these differences, which is easier to do when you are well nourished.

For example, I used to have a hard time controlling my consumption of nuts, and would eat them by the handful. It takes a couple of days to prepare crispy nuts, so we didn't make them all the time. I was OK as long as they weren't around, but whenever they were, I just couldn't help myself. I would have been happy if we had never made them, but the rest of the family enjoyed them, and since nuts are a nutritious food, I had to find a solution that worked for all of us. The compromise we reached was that Mary continued to make them, but they were hidden somewhere in the house where I couldn't see them. As long as they were out of my sight, they were out of my mind and my mouth. This arrangement worked out wonderfully until, mysteriously, I got over my "addiction" to them and was able to eat them without splurging.

Arrangements of this kind require what I call the "three C's": a willingness to Cooperate and Compromise Creatively. Our dilemma with the nuts proves that when you're creative, it's possible to find solutions that benefit everyone.

We've observed that women seem more willing to take steps to improve their health and nutrition than their husbands. Mary is often asked how she was able to get me to a point where I was willing to make a real change. The fact is that we came to the decision independently, and at about the same time, but after our initial decision, Mary helped me in many ways that might be worth sharing for those who have "difficult spouses."

HELPING TO MOTIVATE YOUR HUSBAND

Despite their tough exteriors, men are vulnerable, too, and need as much emotional, spiritual and logistical support as women do. One of the burdens that society places on men is that we are taught from a very young age to never appear weak or in need of help. Consequently, we're often reluctant to ask for help. Sometimes, if help is offered in the wrong way—in the form of accusations, threats or in a tone tainted with pity—it makes us feel weak, resulting in a response that is defensive or even hostile. For a long time, Mary ignored my obesity as completely as my doctors did. She knew I was sensitive to the issue and didn't know how to address it without hurting my feelings. Her solution was to approach the issue in a manner that I was more receptive to.

I am a goal-oriented person who likes to apply logic and reason to problems. Mary eventually came to understand this trait and approached my weight problem as if it were any other mechanical problem, one with a logical solution. She engaged her medical background and focused on the physiological underpinnings of obesity. The human body is in many ways like a machine, just much more complex. By addressing the problem this way, without any fuzzy emotional baggage, I was much more motivated toward finding a solution, because like most men, I tend to view solutions as a product of logic and reason rather than emotion. From this starting point, I could then delve into the deeper, and sometimes more painful, emotional factors that contributed to my health problems.

Mary was a real partner in my effort to change my behavior and reclaim my health. She never made me feel guilty when I felt like giving up. When I accused her of not being there for me, she did not respond with bitterness as she might have in the past, but instead replied with composure and the kind of reason that I could only respect. By treating me in this manner, she made it easier for me to treat her in kind. I was finally able to resist the urge I always had to solve her problems for her—in five minutes or less—and could turn off my analytical mind and just listen to what she had to say. Often she had already reached a solution, and just needed me to listen and perhaps share the burden of a difficult decision.

Cooking was one of the most powerful motivators Mary employed to help me succeed. For a long time, very little cooking had gone on in our house. We mostly frequented restaurants, ate take-out food, ordered pizza, or thawed and reheated pre-cooked frozen foods. When Mary did cook, it was often done with such careless execution that the dish itself became a gustatory proclamation of her disdain for cooking.

For example, if we were short a few ingredients for a dish, she would make it anyway, without any concern for the quality of the end product. Once she substituted parsley for cilantro in my favorite salsa recipe, because, as she explained, "they're both green." On another occasion, she discovered a recipe for goulash whose ingredients included frozen vegetables, ground beef and barbecue sauce. Since the meat was the only ingredient that had to be cooked, it was an easy dish to make. As it turned out, too easy. She served it every night for two weeks until the entire family threatened to run away from home.

But once she discovered real food and real cooking, our home and our palates were transformed. After work, I was no longer tempted to pull into a fast food drive-thru to get something to eat before going home to dinner. Each new day brought with it the tantalizing tastes and smells of real food cooked from scratch. I started calling home an hour or so before leaving work to inquire about the evening's meal, like a kid asking Santa Claus for a sneak peak at his presents. It wasn't just the fact that the food was delicious—it was also doing me a lot of good. In a very short time, I noticed that I felt better, my clothes fit better, I was stronger, and the aches and pains that I woke up with every morning were disappearing. Mary was changing, too. She smiled more often, and seemed more alive than she had been even before we were married. My oldest daughter, who had been steadily gaining weight, was now losing weight, and my youngest, who suffered from frightful mood swings, had been transformed into a little angel.

Even though she was the full-time manager of our home, Mary somehow found the time to cook as well. It sounds impossible, I know, but she was able to do all this because the food changed her as much as it changed me. She was stronger, happier and, for the first time in her life, free of the depression that had clouded her spirit for so many years.

Likewise, I, too took my turn in the kitchen and found that the only thing more enjoyable than eating a wonderful meal is preparing one for the people you love.

WHAT ABOUT THE CHILDREN?

In the case of children, I'm in favor of a governmental model akin to a benign dictatorship. I believe democracy is fine up to a point, but if children were mature enough to make all their own decisions, they wouldn't be children anymore. As parents, my wife and I knew we were failing our children nutritionally. It took years for us to change, but change we did, and once we did, we insisted on the same approach to food for our children.

Because we've been in the same boat, it doesn't surprise us when we hear parents complain that they simply have to buy certain foods, usually junk food, for the kids, because they won't eat anything else. Just like we used to, they buy sub-standard, high-calorie, low-nutrient foods for their children, even though they know these foods will ultimately have a negative impact on their children's health, perhaps for the rest of their lives.

I've sat in the lobby of the movie house waiting for the next showing and watched parents buy their children diabetes starter kits—sticky soda, stale popcorn loaded with rancid soybean oil and fake butter flavoring, trans fat-laden chips and gooey, tooth-rotting, mood-altering candy, all full of artificial flavors, additives and preservatives.

For years, out of ignorance and because of our own addiction to junk food, my wife and I were guilty of the same conduct, but not any more. On the rare occasions when we go to the movies with our children, we bring our own popcorn flavored with real butter. We bring raisins as well as crispy nuts. We also bring cheese, fresh or dried apples, homemade beef jerky or homemade cookies. More often, we rent a movie and watch it at home. That way, it's even easier to eat healthy snacks.

It is the poor diet and lifestyle of parents that leave them so fragile and vulnerable, to the point they are willing to sacrifice their children's health by buying them what I call "shut up" food, just so they can have a little peace and quiet. The good news is that it is never too late to change. Mary and I found that when we improved our diet, we were less irritable and had a lot more patience. We found we were better able to put up with the sometimes difficult behavior of our children—and of each other. Our children have bounced back wonderfully, and so have we.

STEP 4: CREATE HARMONY IN YOUR LIFE

If you've ever been to a concert and listened to the orchestra warm up, you know what a disagreeable cacophony that can be. Imagine trying to concentrate on something important with that noise ringing in your ear. Now imagine how difficult it can be to develop healthier habits for someone distracted by the "noise" of out-of-control debt, a bad relationship or career problems.

The idea that you can make positive change in one area while the rest of your life is a disaster is nonsense. It may be possible for someone with immense willpower, but for most of us, the greater the sum of all our troubles, the more difficult it is to resolve any one of those troubles. Have you ever wondered why, after breaking up with someone you've been close to, that person can seem more appealing and attractive than ever? This is due to our natural inclination to desire the things that are least attainable, but it is also due to the fact that once the stress of a bad relationship has been removed, people find they are able to get back to living again.

Maybe debt and financial problems are adding to your health and nutritional troubles. In a worst-case scenario, where debt collectors are stalking you at home and the office, the stress can wear you down and drive you to indulge in food that will only make your health problems worse. The solution is to take stock of your life and make an honest list of the things you want to change. Prioritize that list, then attack each item in turn. Mounting debt and an unfulfilling career were two of the stresses that contributed to our poor health. But we created a plan, paid off our debts and changed our careers. With that weight lifted from our shoulders, getting the weight off our middles was considerably easier.

Your life is an orchestra. To realize the beautiful music that you're capable of living, you've got to get each section—the percussion, wind instruments and the strings—your debts, relationships and career sections—playing the same song.

STEP 5: SIMPLIFY YOUR LIFE

My older daughter used to play soccer in a junior league. Once, at one of the games, Mary met a woman who wasn't enjoying the game at all—in fact she seemed to be on the verge of a nervous breakdown Her daughter played soccer, but she also had a son who was playing on another soccer team at the same time some distance away. The poor woman had been driving back and forth between games so that she could attend both.

I've known many parents with children enrolled in several extracurricular activities, which all require chauffeuring, team practices, and the outlay of money. These parents have jobs, attend church services and keep other regular appointments—with orthodontists, pediatricians, allergy specialists, psychiatrists, learning specialists—two or three times a week. When your life is this crazy, it is impossible to cook, exercise and get enough sleep. The solution to this dilemma is not to ask, "How do I manage my crazy life?" but to apply the Socratic method and ask, "Do I need this crazy life?" Very often the answer is "no" because what children want most from their parents is not horseback riding lessons, but their time and attention. Enriching your child's life is a wonderful goal, but it should not be at the expense of your sanity.

In 2004, we turned off our television set for good. My frustration with television had been building since the decline of free, over-the-air reception and the steady rise in cable fees. I was offended by the mindless vulgarity of the programming—and that was just the children's shows— and also by the endless messages telling us we should spend all our money on the paycheck-absorbing products and services frequently advertised.

In George Orwell's novel, *1984*, the principal character lives in a world governed by an oppressive regime where two-way televisions called telescreens are installed in every home. These screens are monitored by Big Brother, and they provide a means for the government to broadcast the party line and thus reinforce state-sanctioned "groupthink." In Orwell's world, diversity of opinion is not tolerated.

Television in the real world has a similar power to propagate groupthink and shape public opinion by limiting access to alternative views. Of course, the same can be said of other traditional media: radio, newspapers and magazines, as well as the newest medium, the Internet. But television, through its ubiquity and raw visceral power to command our attention, is unlike anything else in our history.

When our cable service was finally disconnected, the peaceful sound of silence descended into our lives. Raven, the youngest member of our family and the one most susceptible to the siren song of television, began spending more of her free time reading and drawing. We also noted that her RTM (Requests for Toys per Minute) and her RFM (Requests For McDonald's) dropped significantly after the screen went black. Stephanie, our older daughter, who somehow was born with a natural immunity to television, used what little time she had formerly allotted to TV for reading. Mary used her newly found time to reconnect with out-of-state family members, to cook and read, and to apply her medical background to the study of human nutrition and food metabolism.

Of all the changes wrought by our new-found freedom from TV, mine was the most astonishing. I had long complained about my lack of time; now I found myself with a surplus. Suddenly there was all the time in the world to do the things I needed to do, which included focusing more on my health.

Auto retailers are the chief advertisers on TV. I had planned for some time to buy a new car, but without the constant drone of "buy, buy, buy" in my mind, I suddenly saw the superior logic of simply repairing the old car. I did not realize how much my purchasing decisions had been affected by television.

By letting go of some of the trappings of consumerism, we came to discover what was really important. One of the most interesting and pleasant outcomes of these changes was that by ignoring the "call of the mall," we found ourselves with a surplus of income at the end of every month.

STEP 6: EAT AS THOUGH YOUR LIFE DEPENDED ON IT

The junk-food sectors of the food industry have spent billions to convince us to buy more and eat more. We have been told that it absolutely does not matter what we put into our mouths as long as we eat in moderation and, of course, get plenty of physical exercise. Most of us have bought into this lie and many have paid a heavy price for following this advice. Processed foods not only make us fat, they are literally killing us. The main message of this book is to stop eating processed food and to do your own cooking. Do this life as though your life—and your family's life—depended on it . . . because it does.

STEP 7: MAKE EXERCISE PART OF YOUR LIFE

No one has to be convinced that exercise is important. The problem has always been how to make regular exercise a habit. Exercise, like almost everything else, can only become a habit if we take some pleasure in it. I found that my low-energy diet sapped my ability to enjoy exercise.

The chief irony of the lowfat paradigm is embedded in the oft-repeated advice to eat less and exercise more. That makes as much sense as advising someone to put less gas in their car while expecting them to drive farther. This upside-down logic has been the bane of dieters for decades. My experience has led me to the following conclusions about exercise:

- I adopted a flexible energy-dense diet that satisfied my energy needs. When I'm going on a five-mile hike, I know I need more energy than when I'm sitting at my desk in the office, so what I eat changes to reflect my activity.
- I built diversity into my exercise sessions. If you like running, try biking or hiking as well. Alternate between aerobic workouts and anaerobic ones like resistance training.
- If you're new to exercise, get help from a knowledgeable friend or a professional trainer. Trainers can be really affordable.
- I listen to my body and take time off whenever I feel like I need a rest. Don't overwork yourself. Injuries can be painful, time-consuming and can even interrupt your routine for extended periods.
- Look for opportunities to make exercise a practical part of your life. My two-hour-long walking sessions with Mary have more to do with building our relationship and addressing business issues than they do with exercise, but it is great that we can have a business meeting and get a workout, too.

STEP 8: GET HIGH-QUALITY SLEEP

When my weight was in excess of four hundred pounds, getting a good night's sleep was just about impossible. I could only lie down easily on my back. Because of sleep apnea, most mornings I woke up as tired as I had been the night before. I often stayed up until the early hours of the morning, watching television or surfing the web—anything to delay going to bed.

Mary and I had busy schedules, so after changing our diets, we decided that if we were going to find the time to exercise, we would have to get up earlier in the mornings. We began going to bed at nine o'clock so that we could wake up by four in the morning. This was actually easy to do because of our energizing diet. This was the beginning of what has become a habit for us, a habit we love.

It took awhile before I made the connection between sleep and how much better I felt. I realized it wasn't just because I was getting enough sleep, but also because I was sleeping on a regular schedule. Babies intuitively understand the importance of this principle. Recent news stories suggest that medical researchers are beginning to understand it, too.

STEP 9: FIND YOUR MOTIVATION

Besides being a worthwhile personal goal, improving your health is an empowering experience. If this were my only goal, however, I think I would get bored very quickly. Being healthy for the sake of being healthy just isn't enough, but being healthy for the sake of a worthwhile goal provides real motivation. As a species, humans are engineered to test themselves against the world they live in and to seek those goals that seem unreachable. I guess this is why some men climb mountains and why some women fly into space.

Your goals provide the motivation that helps you maintain your commitment. Without goals, the desire to push on when you feel like quitting is diminished. Figure out what you want to do with your life. Don't be shy. You can start a business, get an education or work up the nerve to introduce yourself to the man or woman you want to spend the rest of your life with. Whatever your goals, recognize them, name them and start planning to achieve them.

STEP 10: SHARE WHAT YOU'VE LEARNED

Half the fun of learning how to live a life full of passion is in helping others do the same. When the time comes, share what you know and, as your only compensation, ask them, when they are ready, to do the same for someone else.

Chapter Seventeen

Some Frequently Asked Questions
I'm glad you asked that

The following is a short list of questions that come up regularly. The answers cover some of the important things we learned in our efforts to improve our knowledge about food, weight loss and nutrition.

CREDENTIALS?

Question: What are your credentials?

Answer: I have more than ten years' experience under my belt— no pun intended—as a fat man. For almost thirty years I was an unwilling participant in one of the longest running medical trials to date: the Lowfat Lifestyle trial, which began in the mid-seventies and continues today. I also participated in the High Fructose Corn Syrup trial, which began at about the same time.

I've been in the trenches. I've lived the disastrous results of our failed nutrition policy. I've lost friends and family members to this policy. The suggestion behind the "credentials" question is, "How dare you presume to challenge the status quo of medical orthodoxy?" I dare without apology, and so should anyone else who has found nothing but failure in the policy we now have.

Anyone who can read is free to learn as much as they want to learn. Access to knowledge and the ability to form our own opinions is a right guaranteed to all citizens. I cannot think of a more appropriate application of those immortal words, "Life, liberty and the pursuit of happiness," than to the pursuit of better health.

GOOD AND BAD FOODS?

Question: I've heard it said that there are no good or bad foods, just poor choices. Isn't that right?

Answer: Some health experts are very fond of this idea. They claim that any food can be part of a healthy diet. When they use the phrase "poor choices," they refer to the quantity of the food you eat, not its quality.

The injury wrought by certain foods will vary across a population group based on the relative fitness of each individual. Thus, a small child whose body has yet to be ravaged by decades of poor eating might have a higher tolerance for soda than his father, a forty-five-year-old type-2 diabetic. Does this mean that it's OK for the child to take up soda as a lifelong habit, perhaps with the possibility of becoming a diabetic like his dad, or should he avoid soda altogether in favor of something healthy, like raw milk? Many experts are loath to come right out and say that some foods are worthless and that we do ourselves more harm than good by consuming them, even in moderation.

When I began to be honest with myself, I realized there were certain foods that were absolutely bad for me in the following ways:

- Eating even a moderate amount of these foods made me want more and kept my cravings at a high level.
- They were high-calorie, low-nutrient foods that exerted a cumulatively negative load on my body. Refined sugar was the worst.
- Even a small portion of some foods had an immediate and negative impact on my health. Ultra-pasteurized milk made me violently ill, and MSG gave me headaches.
- They negatively affected me emotionally. Sugar substitutes and a vegetarian diet left me irritable and ill-tempered.
- They satisfied my taste, but not my need. Soy products can

be engineered to taste like real food, but they always left me unsatisfied and fueled my desire to eat more.

- They were killing me.

I realized it just made sense to eliminate these foods from my diet completely, because they were part of the problem. No one would suggest that an alcoholic learn to drink in moderation. Why do we reinforce the bad habits of people addicted to processed food by encouraging them to continue eating the very foods that are at the root of their problem? In truth, the only true beneficiaries of this myth are food manufacturers and retailers.

LIVING WITHOUT FAVORITE FOODS?

Question: Whole foods sound good, but I could never live without my favorite foods. How did you do it?

Answer: I don't live without my favorite foods because I eat everything I want to eat. The most difficult thing for me to grasp was the fact that my tastes and preferences would change. For example, I did not think I could ever live without commercial potato chips, but now I no longer crave them.

The food I eat satisfies me completely. I no longer want or need any of the processed bilge I used to eat. As for comfort foods, I like ice cream, ginger ale, pizza and even candy now and then. I eat all of these things. The difference is that they're all homemade, they contain no additives and they're made with real food, including natural sweeteners. And because the foods I eat are satisfying, I can eat them in moderation.

DEPRIVATION?

Question: Isn't it wrong to deprive yourself of your favorite foods?

Answer: Food industry propagandists and their supporters in the medical field are quite fond of the don't-deprive-yourself-or-you'll-develop-an-obsession school of thought. They even have the studies to prove it. I find it interesting that no one believes that depriving yourself of bashing your neighbor on the head, no matter how much you might want to, will somehow lead to a career as a mugger. And yet, they claim that not letting your children drink soda today will cause them to swill gallons of the stuff when they're older.

The problem is that people really don't understand the nature of deprivation. Simply put, you cannot be deprived of something you do not desire. I found that lowfat fake food diets were all about deprivation, because they kept me in a constant state of desire for something more fulfilling. Once I switched to a balanced diet of whole foods, I was satisfied. Once I was satisfied, my desire for processed foods ended. No desire, no deprivation.

LOSING WEIGHT ON CONVENIENCE FOODS?

Question: I saw a study that proved you can lose weight eating nothing but convenience food. Doesn't that invalidate your argument about convenience foods?

Answer: If you look hard enough, you can find a study that will support any hypothesis you can cook up. This is because studies can easily be engineered to produce any results the researchers want. Many studies are funded by parties with a vested interest in a given outcome. Most people would call this a conflict of interest, but in the strange world of medical research, it is looked on as business as usual.

Unscrupulous researchers can make a study "dance" in a number of ways. I'll list just a few here:

- If you're testing a drug that will be administered to sick people, give it to the healthiest "sick" people you can find and give the placebo to the sickest sick people you can find, to ensure that the study results will be positive.
- If the results of the study at twelve months are disastrous, pretend the study lasted only six months and report those results instead.
- Obscure the results of a study by focusing on relative risk (which

. . . .

makes the differences seem large) while downplaying the absolute risks. In other words, report study results in percentages rather than absolute numbers. For example, if Joe hits Larry two times with a cricket bat before being dosed with a new anti-aggression drug, but only hits Larry one time after being dosed, we can report a fifty percent reduction in aggressive behavior—an impressive dose response indeed. Never mind that we're only talking about two data points. Further, if Joe falls over from a heart attack due to an unintended side effect of the drug, simply bury that small fact somewhere in the study as a "statistically insignificant event."

- Lie.
- If a trial does not produce the desired result, don't publish it.

DOES GOOD FOOD COST MORE?

Question: Doesn't eating better quality food cost more?

Answer: Yes, if you only look at the amount you pay at the checkout counter. Too often we focus on the near-term cost of food while ignoring the long-term consequences. A lifetime of eating nutrient-poor foods along with cheap, lowfat dairy and egg substitutes sapped the strength from both my body and my wallet.

Over the long term, I paid a high price for junk food in prescription and over-the-counter medicines and missed days from work, while suffering a diminished quality of life.

CALORIES IN, CALORIES OUT?

Question: Isn't weight management simply a matter of calories in, calories out?

Answer: If it were that simple, losing weight would be easy. Just cut back on the number of calories consumed, and you'll magically lose weight. Of course, most experienced dieters know that losing weight is anything but simple. In the real world, when you cut back on calories, you get hungry. When you remain in this state for an extended period, you're more likely to binge eat. Cutting back too much on calories can trigger a "starvation" signal to the body to conserve energy—namely fat—so you can't lose weight no matter how little you eat.

A lot of the nutritional advice for maintaining an appropriate weight is based on quantity. We're told we can eat all the vegetables we want, but for everything else, we are advised to limit the amount and balance the intake against what we expend in exercise.

The problem with this advice is that it is oversimplified and thus useless for most people. In my case, it simply did not work. Few of us know how many calories we actually expend walking up a flight of stairs, watching TV or running five miles. If we don't know how many calories we're burning, how can we possibly know how many calories to consume? Furthermore, the calories in-calories out equation ignores the importance of food quality. Eating low-quality foods will work against your efforts to be healthy. In my case, they prevented me from losing weight successfully.

What I eventually discovered was that the type of food I ate could trigger weight loss or weight gain. I learned that some foods affected me emotionally, making me irritable, while other foods left me so fatigued that I was often too tired to exercise. Finally, when I ate low-quality foods my body really didn't like the idea of losing weight and would adapt to increased exercise with an increase in energy conservation. This is why the same amount and type of exercise that would work for me at first stopped working for me six months later. Why health experts continue to ignore these complicating factors of the calories in-calories out equation remains a mystery to me, even today.

HIGH-CARB, LOWFAT?

Question: I heard that for weight loss, a balanced diet should consist of about fifty-five to sixty percent carbohydrates, and be low in fat. Is this a good strategy for losing weight and staying healthy?

Answer: I found this to be true only if my dieting strategy was to get really, really, fat.

I grew up in the era of the four food groups, later replaced by the food pyramid. Carbohydrates are prominently positioned in the pyramid, sending the message that we should eat more of them, so I was shocked when I discovered that livestock producers place pigs and cows on high-carbohydrate diets to fatten them up.

Conversely, increasing the percentage of the right kind of fat in my diet resulted in a corresponding decrease in body weight. No one ever told me that carbohydrates, along with protein, can be converted into stored body fat. The message that all dietary fat equals body fat was a lie I believed for years—even after I cut fat consumption drastically but continued to gain weight.

In truth, such a diet might work for helping some people lose weight, but if you've been following the lowfat advice and it hasn't worked for you, it might be wise to consider the alternatives. Additionally, and separate from the issue of losing weight, we have to ask whether a plant-based, processed-food diet is healthy. When we consider the relentless increase of heart disease and cancer in this country, it certainly should make us wonder whether the diet prescribed by doctors and nutritional experts might be a contributing factor.

FRUIT JUICE A HEALTHY ALTERNATIVE?

Question: Aren't fruit juices a healthy alternative to sodas?

Answer: Fruits contain a simple sugar called fructose. For a time, I actually believed that fruit juice was a diet drink, dutifully consuming large quantities of juice after exercising. Even though the juices were very sweet, I didn't think of them as a source of "sugar." Sugar was a white granular substance that came in a bag from the grocery store. Fruit juice was "natural," I reasoned. I believed that as long as I was careful about my consumption of white sugar, I could drink fruit juice to my heart's content. I had no idea how much sugar I was consuming in the form of juices, as well as just about every convenience food I purchased. Most of them contain some form of added sugar, often in the form of high fructose corn syrup. Because the dietary experts spent so much time emphasizing dietary fat as the source of my obesity, I ignored the mountains of sugar that were hidden in everything I consumed, from tomato sauce to "healthy" cereals.

DOES FAT MAKE YOU FAT?

Question: Eating fat makes you fat, right?

Answer: Maybe, maybe not. Our bodies use glucose for energy. Most of that energy comes in the form of sugars and starches from plant sources such as fruits, vegetables and grains. Milk is the only animal food that contains sugar; the type of sugar in milk is called lactose. What is less well known is the fact that our bodies can utilize fat as an energy source as well.

I found that when I was consuming dietary fat along with the sugar, starches and grains that comprised the bulk of my diet, I gained weight. Like most people, I assumed it was the fat in my diet that was making me fat. When I began eating a more balanced diet of traditional foods, one that reduced the amounts of sugar, starch, grains and processed foods, I discovered I could eat fat—the right fats—and still lose weight.

ASKING MY DOCTOR?

Question: What's wrong with asking my doctor about how to lose weight?

Answer: Nothing. . . if your doctor is educated in the complexities of nutrition and weight loss. I've had several doctors over the years, and they were all great people, but none of them, not one, could give me any useful advice about weight loss.

The family doctor is great when it comes to the "simple" things, like broken bones, diagnosing an illness based on a predefined list of symptoms, administering physicals and writing prescriptions. They are trained to recognize and deal with acute disease issues and other obvious abnormalities. We would all fare poorly without them. But when it comes to long-term chronic conditions like obesity, the slow killer, they are less helpful and tend to rely on useless advice, such as, "Just stop eating so much."

Simply knowing that a diet high in refined carbohydrates can cause weight gain, while reducing carbs and adding good fats can help people lose weight, goes a long way toward providing obese people with basic advice they can actually use. This isn't quack science. Any decent anatomy or physiology textbook lays out the basics of macronutrient metabolism, but until recent attention focused on how carbohydrates and fats are metabolized in the body, most doctors would have told you the opposite. Many still do.

The fact that many doctors have weight problems of their own highlights the difficulties involved in losing weight. I believe the ideal doctor-patient relationship is one where both parties utilize their strengths to help each other. Patients should make an honest effort to tell the truth about their condition, instead of simply accepting a treatment plan that they know will fail. Doctors should work with their patients to find workable solutions to dietary and nutritional problems, not pretend that they have all the answers.

WHAT ABOUT THIN PEOPLE?

Question: None of this really applies to me since I'm thin, right?

Answer: There's an old saying: "You can never be too rich, too thin or too beautiful." While I agree with the first and last items, I take issue with the second. While it's possible to be thin and healthy, the idea that being thin always equals health is a myth perpetuated by popular culture and the fashion and entertainment industries. I'm no exception to this disease of the mind. I, too, wanted to be thin and assumed that low body weight directly correlated with good health.

When I was a vegetarian, I lost fifty pounds and certainly looked healthier, but I knew that inside it was a different story. I was weak and lacked the strength I once had. I had headaches, was irritable, lacked focus, had digestion problems and felt bad most of the time. I ate lots of fruits and vegetables, kept dietary fat to a minimum, ate soy every day, didn't drink or smoke . . . and I felt awful.

The fallacy that equates thinness with health and beauty is having a tragic effect on a generation of young women who try desperately to emulate the emaciated females they see in the popular media. These poor women drift through their daily lives gaunt and hollow-eyed, with sunken cheeks and pallid skin, in a perpetual state of starvation. Someone needs to tell these waifs that there's nothing sexy about starvation. Their appearance only tells half the story. The rest—what is happening to their bodies on the inside—does not become apparent until later.

Chapter Eighteen

Rebirth
The end is just the beginning

When Mary and I began our journey we had no idea what the outcome would be of one simple idea: changing what we ate.

One of the wonderful results of my transformation is this book. I have always loved to write but for years lacked the courage to take that first step. I thank you, the reader, for making the effort worthwhile by sharing with me a portion of your time. Along with other titles in the works, I've taken my story and my message to the streets in the hope that those people who once thought that the course of their lives was predestined might see that it is possible to change and change on their own terms. I enjoy nothing more than talking to people and encouraging them to visualize a better future for themselves.

Cleaning up my diet cleaned up my body, my mind and my life. I can think more clearly now, and I notice opportunities that I could never have seen before when I was too wrapped up in the physical and emotional problems created and exacerbated by poor health.

My education in the value of traditional foods continues, as do my efforts at self-improvement. Physically, I am free of the aches and pains, sleep apnea, asthma, mild depression and hypertension that once plagued me.

We are big supporters of independent food producers and purchase much of our food from local farmers. We cook virtually all of our meals from scratch. The return on our investment—our improved health—has been nothing short of miraculous. Conversely, our costs for over-the-counter and prescription medicines has been reduced to zero. I haven't had a cold for two years. I'm sharper mentally and my personal zeal for life burns brighter now than it has since my college years. Mary, thankfully free of medication as well, has had a similar experience. We still get up at four in the morning several times a week to take our two-hour walks, when we talk in the quiet hours before sunrise. Each new day for us is a special blessing that we cherish as if it were our last.

Our daughters have experienced a miraculous change as well. They exercise regularly—and are considerably more fit. They know how to read product labels and how to evaluate critically the often dubious health claims about food. They rarely fall ill now but when they do feel under the weather, a good night's rest always solves the problem. We're teaching them how to cook, and we lead by example by making sure we eat a good breakfast, providing real food for lunch, and sitting down together as a family for the evening meal.

It's hard to believe that before my miraculous transformation, I thought my life was over. I find it impossible to convey just how thankful I am for this second chance.

On a walk with my oldest daughter one morning, I asked her what she thought of the many changes her mother and I had made and the challenges we've faced as a family. She thought for a moment and replied, "We're happier now."

She was right.

Resources
You take if from here

BOOKS

The Second Brain: A Groundbreaking New Understanding of Nervous Disorders of the Stomach and Intestine, by Michael Gershon.

Nourishing Traditions: The Cookbook that Challenges Politically Correct Nutrition and the Diet Dictocrats, by Sally Fallon with Mary G. Enig, PhD.

Safe Food: Bacteria, Biotechnology, and Bioterrorism, by Marion Nestle.

Food Politics: How the Food Industry Influences Nutrition and Health, by Marion Nestle.

Fast Food Nation: The Dark Side of the All-American Meal, by Eric Schlosser.

Fat Land: How Americans Became the Fattest People in the World, by Greg Critser.

The Cholesterol Myths: Exposing the Fallacy that Saturated Fat and Cholesterol Cause Heart Disease, by Uffe Ravnskov, MD, PhD.

Know Your Fats: The Complete Primer for Understanding the Nutrition of Fats, Oils and Cholesterol, by Mary G. Enig, PhD.

The Hungry Gene: The Inside Story of the Obesity Industry, by Ellen Ruppel Shell.

RESOURCES

Eat Fat, Lose Fat, by Mary Enig, PhD and Sally Fallon.

A Consumer's Dictionary of Food Additives, by Ruth Winter, MS.

The Whole Soy Story: The dark side of America's favorite health food, by Kaayla T. Daniel, PhD, CCN.

ARTICLES
"The Soft Science of Dietary Fat," *Journal of Science* (March 30, 2001, Volume 291, pages 2536-2545), www.sciencemag.org.

WEBSITES

The Weston A. Price Foundation: www.westonaprice.org.

The Omnivore: www.theomnivore.com.

The International Network of Cholesterol Skeptics: www.thincs.org.

A Campaign for Real Milk: www.realmilk.com.

The Healthy Alternative to Trans Fats: www.eatfastlosefat.com.

MSG Dangers: www.truthinlabeling.org.

Index

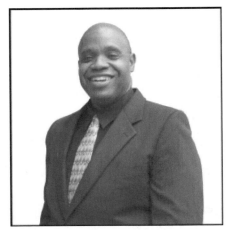

Richard Morris is a writer, publisher, real food activist, health researcher, speaker and self-described nutrition contrarian. An ardent supporter of fair trade for the family farm, Richard is the creator and chief instigator of BreadandMoney.com, a web site that describes the virtues of traditional foods and suburban homesteading.

To arrange a speaking
engagement for your group,
or to provide feedback
on this book,
write to Richard at
feedback@breadandmoney.com
or send a letter to
P.O. Box 2452
Woodbridge, VA 22195